# Ulcerative Colitis Cookbook

600+ Healthy, Tasty & Delicious Gut-Friendly Recipes to Restore Your Body and Relieve the Symptoms of Ulcerative Colitis Fastly

## Louise Acosta

# TABLE OF CONTENTS

# INTRODUCTION

A good resource is essential for studying and discovering the topics you are curious about. This is available to everyone, not just those with ulcerative colitis problems. Those who have not yet received a diagnosis have the chance to learn more about their bodies and how to take the best possible care of them. The goal of this cookbook is to provide readers with a tool that will instruct them on how to properly prepare meals for their bodies. The intention behind the dishes and meals is to reduce inflammation and improve intestinal health.

Cuisine options are quite restricted for those who have this illness, so it's crucial to find any food that might improve your health. The majority of foods may cause the illness to flare up and exacerbate its already uncomfortable symptoms.

So you need a diet plan if you want to control ulcerative colitis. You can consume foods that won't aggravate the illness, and it will be best for you if you follow the recommended diet. In fact, you should find out what meals might make the situation more tolerable, since some of them can even make it better. You may locate fantastic eating alternatives with the help of this cookbook, and you'll see the difference. You'll discover that your symptoms can be controlled and that your overall health has improved. You may use it to examine your alternatives and choose which is best for you.

## Knowledge of Ulcerative Colitis

An overactive immune system that begins attacking your own body is what leads to ulcerative colitis. Inflammation of the colon lining is the first sign. If this is left untreated, the inflammation leads to the development of tiny open sores and ulcers on your colon's lining.

Inflammation is the first stage of the ulcerative colitis process for some individuals. Sadly, we have become so used to seeking the easy solution rather than looking deeper to identify the cause of the issue. Many of us use over-the-counter medicine in this situation to get prompt relief from the stomach discomfort we begin to feel. Even if this band-aid solution only offers temporary relief, the pain and discomfort eventually return, and we continue to take drugs until the situation gets so serious that we decide to see a doctor.

Unfortunately, at this stage, the colon's lining has developed open ulcers and sores as a result of the disease's progression. Once ulcerative colitis has been identified as your condition, you will go through periods when your symptoms are painful and periods when they aren't.

According to the severity of the illnesses and the sorts of therapies you have received, your objective is to remain in a state of remission for as long as you can. This might take anything from a few weeks to several years.

**According to studies, those who are most at risk for developing ulcerative colitis include:**

- Those who are closely related to someone who has IBD of any kind. This person can be a parent, kid, or sibling.
- People in their mid-teenage years, or between the ages of 15 and 30.Although ulcerative colitis is most prevalent in people between the ages of 15 and 30, it is crucial to remember that it may occur at any age.
- Additionally, it seems that ulcerative colitis affects more people of Jewish heritage.

### Signs and Symptoms of Ulcerative Colitis

The most typical signs and symptoms include: frequent diarrhea; an almost insatiable urge to pass stool; bursts of cramping and pain in the stomach; a constant need to pass stool even when you can feel that your stomach is empty; rectal bleeding manifested by blood-stained stool; passing pus or mucus when passing stool; weight loss; nausea; chronic fatigue; and fever.

People with ulcerative colitis have both periods of remission, during which the symptoms entirely subside, and times of flare-ups, during which the aforementioned symptoms appear. Weeks or even years may pass between remissions.

### The origins of ulcerative colitis

Doctors and scientific experts have not been able to identify the precise etiology of ulcerative colitis. However, they believe that the following things may lead to ulcerative colitis:

- Over reactive immune response
- genetics
- Environment
- gut microbiota

## Diet For Ulcerative Colitis

A persistent condition called ulcerative colitis results in inflammation and damage to the colon and rectum. People who have ulcerative colitis often suffer diarrhea and stomach cramps, and when the condition flares up, they may also endure bleeding and discomfort. The quantity of fiber in the diet is often restricted for those who must adhere to a stringent low-residue diet because they have ulcerative colitis.

The waste products that are left over after dietary fiber has been removed from food are referred to as "residue." The fraction of food that cannot be absorbed in the digestive system and is not utilized as energy is referred to as fiber in conventional dietary recommendations. The low-residue diet, on the other hand, excludes dietary fiber and restricts consumption to the leftover waste products. Patients with ulcerative colitis are often told to follow this kind of diet because it limits the amount of fiber they eat. Too much fiber can cause diarrhea and stomach pain.

**The Fundamentals of a Low-Residue Diet**

One should constantly adhere to certain low-residue diet fundamentals. These should be avoided in addition to the items listed above while following a low-residue diet. Let's quickly review these guidelines:

- No more than 10-15 grams of fiber should be included in a low-fiber diet per day.
- Fruits and vegetables, which include some fiber, must be thoroughly cooked.
- Avoid dishes with a lot of seasoning. It's not necessary to cease flavoring the dish altogether. Simply make sure that the seasoning is used sparingly.
- Completely avoid frying and attempt to cook by baking, boiling, broiling, roasting, stewing, microwaving, or creaming instead of eating huge meals since they may induce pain from stomach distention.

The low-residue diet is only utilized for a short period of time or until your digestive system returns to normal. Once things have returned to normal, you may start eating regularly, merely avoiding things you can't usually handle.

## Banana and Pear Pita Pockets

Time to prepare: 10 minutes
Time to cook: 0 minutes
Servings: 1
**Ingredients:**
- 1/2 small banana, peeled & sliced
- 1 round refined white flour pita bread
- 1/2 small pear, peeled, seedless, cored, cooked & sliced
- 1/4 cup low-fat Cottage cheese

**Directions:**
1. In a small bowl, mix the cottage cheese, banana, and pears.
2. Cut a pocket out of your pita bread and fill it with the mixture. Serve.

**Nutritional Info:** Calories: 402; Fat: 2g; Carbs: 87g; Protein: 14g; Fiber: 1g

## French Toast

Time to prepare: 10 minutes
Time to cook: 0 minutes
Servings: 1
**Ingredients:**
- 2 slices of white bread
- 1 egg
- ¼ cup nondairy milk
- 2 tablespoon apple or smooth peanut butter
- 1 tablespoon olive oil
- 2 teaspoon maple syrup
- A pinch of salt & cinnamon

**Directions:**
1. In your bowl, combine the milk, egg, salt, and maple syrup. Bread should be dipped in this mixture on both sides.
2. Both toasts should be browned for two to three minutes on each side in hot oil in a frying pan.
3. Serve with smooth peanut butter or apples on top.

**Nutritional Info:** Calories: 366; Fat: 12.6g; Carbs: 48g; Protein: 11.6g; Fiber: 1.7g

## Ricotta Pear Cream Bowl

Time to prepare: 10 minutes
Time to cook: 0 minutes
Servings: 4
**Ingredients:**
- 1 (15-oz.) container part-skim ricotta cheese
- ½ cup canned pears, drained
- 1 teaspoon fresh lemon juice
- 2-4 drops of liquid stevia

**Directions:**
1. Add all the ingredients to a food processor and process until smooth, excluding the pears.
2. Serve right away.

**Nutritional Info:** Calories: 127; Fat: 6.8g; Carbs: 6.8g; Protein: 9.8g; Fiber: 0.5g

## Cheesy Egg Tomato Bowl

Time to prepare: 10 minutes
Time to cook: 0 minutes
Servings: 3
**Ingredients:**
- 5 hard-boiled eggs, peeled and sliced
- 1/3 cup low-fat cottage cheese
- 1 large tomato, peeled, seeded & chopped
- Salt & ground black pepper to taste

**Directions:**
1. In a bowl, mix the cheese, black pepper, and salt until well combined.
2. Include the egg slices and combine by stirring. Serve after adding tomato slices on top.

**Nutritional Info:** Calories: 131; Fat: 7.8g; Carbs: 2g; Fiber: 0.2g; Protein: 12.9g

## Apple Yogurt Cheese Bowl

Time to prepare: 10 minutes
Time to cook: 0 minutes
Servings: 2

**Ingredients:**
- ½ cup fat-free plain yogurt
- ½ cup low-fat cottage cheese
- 2 teaspoon extra-virgin olive oil
- 1 small apple, peeled, cored, and sliced

**Directions:**
1. Combine the oil, yogurt, cheese, and cinnamon in a sizable bowl.
2. Split the yogurt mixture between two bowls for serving.
3. Add apple slices on top, then serve right away.

**Nutritional Info:** Calories: 157; Fat: 5.9g; Carbs: 13.3g; Fiber: 0.9g; Protein: 13.6g

## Fresh Mashed Banana Porridge

Time to prepare: 10 minutes
Time to cook: 0 minutes
Servings: 4

**Ingredients:**
- 4 small bananas, peeled, sliced, & mashed
- 1 tablespoon low-fat butter softened
- ¼ teaspoon ground cinnamon

**Directions:**
1. In a large bowl, combine the mashed bananas, almond butter, and cinnamon.
2. Stir everything together, then serve right away.

**Nutritional Info:** Calories: 165; Fat: 3.9g; Carbs: 30.7g; Protein: 2g; Fiber: 0.1g

## Baked Simple Eggs

Time to prepare: 5 minutes
Time to cook: 8-12 minutes
Servings: 6

**Ingredients:**
- 12 large eggs
- Salt & ground black pepper to taste

**Directions:**
1. Preheat the oven to 350 degrees Fahrenheit and oil a 12-cup whoopie pie pan.
2. Break an egg in a small bowl, then gently spoon it into the whoopie pie pan's prepared cups. Continue with the remaining eggs.
3. Bake for 8 to 12 minutes, depending on desired doneness. Before serving, season it with salt and black pepper.

**Nutritional Info:** Calories: 143; Fat: 9.9g; Carbs: 0.8g; Protein: 12.6g; Fiber: 0g

## Fried Eggs with Tomatoes

Time to prepare: 10 minutes
Time to cook: 6 minutes
Servings: 2

**Ingredients:**
- 2 tablespoon olive oil
- 2 eggs
- 1 tomato, peeled, seeded & chopped
- Salt & ground black pepper to taste

**Directions:**
1. In your large cast-iron pan, heat the oil over medium heat.
2. Crack an egg into your small bowl, carefully pour it into the pan, and cook within 212–3 minutes, gently tilting the pan occasionally.
Carefully transfer the cooked egg onto a plate. Divide the tomatoes onto each plate with eggs. Sprinkle each egg with salt and black pepper, and serve.

**Nutritional Info:** Calories: 189; Fat: 18.4g; Carbs: 1.6g; Fiber: 0.4g; Protein: 5.8g

## Cheddar Scramble Eggs

Time to prepare: 10 minutes
Time to cook: 8 minutes
Servings: 6

**Ingredients:**
- 2 tablespoon olive oil
- 12 large eggs, beaten lightly
- 4 oz low-fat cheddar cheese, shredded

- Salt & ground black pepper to taste

**Directions:**

1. In your large pan, heat the oil over medium heat.
2. Add the eggs, salt, and black pepper and cook within 3 minutes, stirring continuously.
3. Remove and immediately stir in the cheese. Serve immediately.

**Nutritional Info:** Calories: 242; Fat: 0.5g; Carbs: 27.1g; Fiber: 7.1g; Protein: 17.4g

### Spinach Salmon Scramble

Time to prepare: 10 minutes
Time to cook: 7 minutes
Servings: 3

**Ingredients:**

- 2 cups fresh spinach, chopped finely
- ½ cup cooked salmon, chopped finely
- 4 eggs, beaten
- 1 tablespoon olive oil
- Salt & ground black pepper to taste

**Directions:**

1. Cook the spinach with black pepper in the oil in your skillet for two minutes over high heat.
2. Add the salmon and set the heat to medium. Within 3 to 4 minutes, add the eggs and simmer while stirring constantly. Serve right away.

**Nutritional Info:** Calories: 200, Fat: 14.7g, Carbs: 1.3g, Protein: 15.3g, Fiber: 0.52g

### Basil Tomato Scramble

Time to prepare: 10 minutes
Time to cook: 5 minutes
Servings: 2

**Ingredients:**

- 4 eggs
- ¼ cup fresh basil, chopped
- ½ cup tomatoes, peeled, seeded, and chopped
- 1 tablespoon olive oil

- Salt & ground black pepper to taste

**Directions:**

1. In a large bowl, whisk together the eggs, salt, and black pepper. Stir in the tomatoes and basil after adding them.
2. In a large nonstick skillet over medium-high heat, warm the oil. Within three to five minutes, add the egg mixture and stir-fry. Serve right away.

**Nutritional Info:** Calories: 195; Fat: 15.9g; Carbs: 2.6g; Protein: 11.6g; Fiber: 0.7g

### Mushroom Chives Omelet

Time to prepare: 10 minutes
Time to cook: 25 minutes
Servings: 4

**Ingredients:**

- 6 large eggs
- ½ cup low-fat milk
- 1/3 cup fresh mushrooms, cut into slices
- 1 tablespoon chives, minced
- 1 tablespoon coconut oil
- Sea salt & ground black pepper to taste

**Directions:**

1. Lightly oil a pie plate and preheat the oven to 350°F.
2. In a bowl, combine the eggs, salt, pepper, and coconut oil.
3. Evenly pour the egg mixture into the pie plate that has been prepared. Add the mushroom on top, then evenly distribute the chives.
4. Bake for 20 to 25 minutes, then slice and serve.

**Nutritional Info:** Calories: 125; Fat: 7.8g; Carbs: 3.1g; Protein: 10.8g; Fiber: 0.4g

### Zucchini Tomato Omelet

Time to prepare: 15 minutes
Time to cook: 15 minutes
Servings: 4

**Ingredients:**

- 4 large eggs
- 1 medium zucchini, seeded and cubed
- ½ medium tomato, seeded and chopped
- 2 tablespoon extra-virgin olive oil
- ¼ cup almond milk
- 1 teaspoon salt

**Directions:**

1. In your large non-stick pan, heat the olive oil over moderate heat. Add the zucchini and tomato, then cook for 5 to 10 minutes until they are soft.

2. In a separate bowl, mix the eggs, milk, and salt. Pour the egg mixture into the pan and stir within 5 minutes to cook through, then serve!

**Nutritional Info:** Calories: 160; Fat: 10g; Carbs: 14g; Protein: 6g; Fiber: 2g

## Tomato Omelet

Time to prepare: 10 minutes
Time to cook: 5 minutes
Servings: 2

**Ingredients:**

- 4 large eggs, beaten
- 1 tablespoon olive oil
- ½ cup tomato, peeled, seeded, & chopped
- Pinch of ground black pepper
- Salt to taste

**Directions:**

1. In your cast-iron pan, heat the oil over medium-high heat and cook the tomato for about 1 minute.

2. Add the egg mixture to the pan evenly and cook for about 2 minutes. Carefully tilt the pan and cook for about 2 minutes more.

3. Transfer the omelet to your plate and cut it into two wedges. Serve hot with black pepper and salt.

**Nutritional Info:** Calories: 211; Fat: 17g; Carbs: 2.6g; Protein: 12g; Fiber: 0.6g

## Feta Salmon Omelet

Time to prepare: 10 minutes
Time to cook: 7 minutes
Servings: 2

**Ingredients:**

- 5 eggs
- 2 tablespoon olive oil
- 4 oz smoked salmon, roughly chopped
- 2 tablespoon low-fat feta cheese, crumbled
- Ground black pepper to taste

**Directions:**

1. In a bowl, whisk together the eggs, salt, and black pepper.

2. In a frying pan, heat the oil over medium heat. The beaten eggs should be poured evenly and cooked for 1-2 minutes without stirring.

3. Insert the smoked salmon in the omelet's middle and cook for 40 to 50 seconds. Add the cheese and continue to simmer for two to three minutes. Serve right away.

**Nutritional Info:** Calories: 337; Fat: 27.2g; Carbs: 1.1g; Protein: 22.8g; Fiber: 0g

## Tuna Tomato Omelet

Time to prepare: 10 minutes
Time to cook: 5 minutes
Servings: 2

**Ingredients:**

- 4 eggs
- ¼ cup unsweetened almond milk
- 1 (5-oz.) can of water-packed tuna, drained & flaked
- ½ cup tomato, peeled, seeded & chopped
- ¼ cup low-fat cheddar cheese, shredded
- 1 tablespoon olive oil
- Salt & ground black pepper to taste

**Directions:**

1. Beat the eggs, milk, salt, and black pepper in a bowl. Stir in the tuna after adding it.

2. Heat the oil in a large nonstick frying pan over medium heat. Without stirring, spread the egg mixture out evenly and cook for 1-2 minutes.

3. Place the tomato on top of the egg mixture and top with cheese. Cook under cover for 30 to 60 seconds.

4. Cut the omelet in half, take it out, and serve it right away.

**Nutritional Info:** Calories: 322; Fat: 20.2g; Carbs: 3.1g; Protein: 31.4g; Fiber: 0.5g

### Potato Omelet

Time to prepare: 10 minutes
Time to cook: 15 minutes
Servings: 6
**Ingredients:**
- ¾ lb. potatoes, peeled & sliced thinly
- 6 eggs
- ½ cup olive oil
- Salt & ground black pepper to taste

**Directions:**
1. In your large pan, heat the oil over medium-high heat and cook the potatoes with salt and black pepper for about 6–8 minutes, stirring occasionally.

2. Meanwhile, beat the eggs, salt, and black pepper in a bowl. Add the egg mixture to the pan and gently stir to combine.

3. Adjust the heat to low and cook for about 2–3 minutes, until the eggs begin to set. Carefully flip the omelet and cook for about 1-2 minutes until the eggs are set. Serve hot.

**Nutritional Info:** Calories: 246; Fat: 21.2g; Carbs: 9.3g; Protein: 6.5g; Fiber: 1.3g

### Cheesy Avocado Frittata

Time to prepare: 15 minutes
Time to cook: 12 minutes

Servings: 6
**Ingredients:**
- 8 eggs, beaten well
- 8 tablespoon low-fat milk
- 2 oz feta cheese, crumbled
- ½ cup low-fat mozzarella cheese, grated
- ¼ cup scallion, sliced
- 2 teaspoon olive oil
- 1 large avocado, peeled, pitted, & sliced lengthwise
- Salt & ground black pepper to taste

**Directions:**
1. Preheat the oven's broiler, and arrange the oven rack about 4–5 inches from the heating element.

2. Beat the eggs, milk, salt, and black pepper in a bowl.

3. Heat the oil in your heavy oven-proof frying skillet over medium-low heat. Add the egg mixture and cook for about 2 minutes.

4. Add the mozzarella and scallion and cook for about 5 minutes. Arrange the avocado slices over the egg mixture and sprinkle with the feta cheese.

5. Cover and cook for about 3 minutes. Remove the lid, transfer the skillet into the oven, and broil for about 2 minutes. Serve hot.

**Nutritional Info:** Calories: 195; Fat: 14.6g; Carbs: 4.32g; Protein: 12.5g; Fiber: 1.55g

### Tomato Asparagus Frittata

Time to prepare: 15 minutes
Time to cook: 16 minutes
Servings: 2
**Ingredients:**
- 5 trimmed asparagus spears
- 5 cherry tomatoes
- 3 eggs
- 1 tablespoon extra-virgin olive oil
- 1/2 tablespoon chopped fresh thyme

- 1/4 teaspoon sea salt
- A pinch of freshly ground black pepper

**Directions:**
1. Set the broiler to its maximum temperature.
2. In a large ovenproof skillet, heat the olive oil to medium-high heat. Add the asparagus and simmer for 5 minutes while stirring.
3. Add the tomatoes and simmer for 3 minutes, occasionally stirring.
4. In a larger bowl, combine the thyme, salt, eggs, and pepper. Pour slowly over the asparagus and tomatoes.
5. Adjust the heat to medium and cook the eggs for 3 minutes, or until they are set. Cook the dish until puffed and browned in 3–5 minutes under the broiler. Serve!

**Nutritional Info:** Calories: 172; Fat: 13.5g; Carbs: 3.5g; Protein: 9.4g; Fiber: 1.2g

## Zucchini Frittata

Time to prepare: 10 minutes
Time to cook: 18 minutes
Servings: 6
**Ingredients:**
- 2 medium zucchinis, peeled, seeded & cut into ¼-inch thick round slices
- 8 eggs
- ½ cup low-fat feta cheese, crumbled
- 2 tablespoon unsweetened almond milk
- 1 tablespoon olive oil
- Salt & ground black pepper to taste

**Directions:**
1. Set the oven to 350°F.
2. Thoroughly combine the milk, eggs, salt, and pepper in a bowl. Place aside.
3. Cook the zucchini for around 5 minutes in the oil that has been heated over medium heat in an ovenproof pan. Stir for approximately a minute after adding the egg mixture. Evenly distribute the cheese over the top.
4. Place the pan in the oven, and bake the eggs for 10 to 12 minutes, or until they are set. Serve after cutting into desired-sized wedges.

**Nutritional Info:** Calories: 149; Fat: 11g; Carbs: 3.4g; Protein: 10g; Fiber: 0.8g

## Mushroom & Spinach Frittata

Time to prepare: 10 minutes
Time to cook: 33 minutes
Servings: 5
**Ingredients:**
- 1 cup canned mushrooms, drained and chopped
- 1½ cup fresh spinach, chopped
- 8 eggs
- ½ cup unsweetened almond milk
- 1 tablespoon olive oil
- Salt & ground black pepper to taste

**Directions:**
1. Set the oven to 350°F.
2. Beat the eggs, milk, salt, and black pepper in a large basin. Place aside.
3. Cook the mushrooms for around 5 to 6 minutes in the oil that has been heated over medium heat in your big ovenproof pan. Cook the spinach for 2 to 3 minutes after adding it.
4. Evenly distribute the egg mixture over the top and simmer for 4 minutes without stirring.
5. Place the pan in the oven and bake for 12 to 15 minutes, depending on how done you want it. Serve after cutting into desired-sized wedges.

**Nutritional Info:** Calories: 134; Fat: 10.2g; Carbs: 1.5g; Protein: 9.7g; Fiber: 0.4g

## Zucchini & Spinach Frittata

Time to prepare: 10 minutes
Time to cook: 20 minutes
Servings: 4

**Ingredients:**
- 6 eggs
- 2 cups fresh baby spinach, chopped
- ¾ cup zucchini, peeled, seeded, and chopped
- ½ cup unsweetened almond milk
- ¼ cup fresh cilantro, chopped
- Salt & ground black pepper to taste

**Directions:**

1. Preheat the oven to 400°F, then gently butter a pie plate.

2. Combine the eggs, milk, salt, and black pepper in a large bowl. Place aside.

3. Combine the zucchini and cilantro in a separate bowl.

4. Evenly distribute the zucchini mixture in the prepared pie plate, then top with the egg mixture.

5. Bake for 20 minutes, let cool, then cut into wedges of the appropriate size and serve hot.

**Nutritional Info:** Calories: 106; Fat: 7.1g; Carbs: 2.1g; Protein: 9.1g; Fiber: 0.7g

### Potato & Zucchini Frittata

Time to prepare: 10 minutes
Time to cook: 26 minutes
Servings: 6

**Ingredients:**
- 8 eggs
- 1 large potato, peeled & cut into thin slices
- 2 zucchinis, peeled, seeded & sliced
- 2 tablespoon olive oil
- Salt & ground black pepper to taste

**Directions:**

1. Heat the oil over medium-low heat in a big ovenproof pan. Simmer the potato for 7-8 minutes after adding it. After adding the zucchini, sauté it for three to four minutes.

2. In the meantime, combine the eggs, salt, and pepper in a bowl. Spread this mixture evenly over the vegetables, turn the heat to low, and simmer for a further 10 minutes to complete.

3. Place the pan in the broiler for 3–4 minutes, or until the top is golden brown. Serve.

**Nutritional Info:** Calories: 156; Fat: 10.7g; Carbs: 7.6g; Protein: 8.7g; Fiber: 1.3g

### Carrot Zucchini Frittata

Time to prepare: 10 minutes
Time to cook: 20 minutes
Servings: 2

**Ingredients:**
- 2 eggs, beaten
- 2 boiled potatoes, peeled & mashed
- ½ cup carrot, peeled & shredded
- ½ cup zucchini, peeled, seeded & shredded
- ½ cup soft cheese, crumbled
- 2 tablespoon olive oil
- ½ teaspoon salt

**Directions:**

1. Set the oven to 375 degrees.

2. In your saucepan, heat the oil before adding the vegetables. Cook for two to three minutes, then remove and let cool.

3. Apply olive oil to the baking dish. Spread the eggs and vegetables out and sprinkle salt over them. 10 to 12 minutes of baking

4. Take out, top with cheese, and bake for an additional 4-5 minutes, or until the cheese has melted. Serve!

**Nutritional Info:** Calories: 338; Fat: 16.9g; Carbs: 36.5g; Protein: 8.7g; Fiber: 2.3g

### Chicken Asparagus Tomato Frittata

Time to prepare: 10 minutes
Time to cook: 12 minutes
Servings: 4

**Ingredients:**
- 6 eggs, beaten lightly
- ½ cup cooked chicken, chopped

- 1/3 cup boiled asparagus, chopped
- 1/3 cup low-fat Parmesan cheese, grated
- ¼ cup tomatoes, peeled, seeded & chopped
- ¼ cup part-skim mozzarella cheese, shredded
- Salt & ground black pepper to taste

**Directions:**

1. Pre-heat the broiler of your oven.
2. In a bowl, beat the Parmesan cheese, eggs, salt, and black pepper.
3. In a large ovenproof pan, melt the butter over medium-high heat and cook the chicken and asparagus for about 2–3 minutes.
4. Add the egg mixture and tomatoes and stir to combine. Cook for about 4–5 minutes. Remove and sprinkle with the mozzarella cheese.
5. Transfer the pan under the broiler and broil for about 3–4 minutes, until slightly puffed. Cut into desired-sized wedges and serve immediately.

**Nutritional Info:** Calories: 158; Fat: 7.3g; Carbs: 1.7g; Protein: 16.8g; Fiber: 0.4g

### Cheesy Chicken Spinach Frittata

Time to prepare: 10 minutes
Time to cook: 43 minutes
Servings: 8

**Ingredients:**

- 4 large egg whites
- 2 large eggs
- 4 cups fresh spinach, chopped
- 2 cups cooked chicken, chopped
- 1¼ cup unsweetened almond milk
- 1 cup low-fat cheddar cheese, shredded
- 1 tablespoon low-fat Parmesan cheese, shredded
- 1 teaspoon olive oil
- Salt & ground black pepper to taste

**Directions:**

1. Warm your oven to 350oF and grease a 9-inch pie plate.
2. In your pan, heat the oil over medium heat and cook the spinach for about 2–3 minutes. Stir in the chicken and transfer the mixture into the prepared pie dish evenly.
3. Add the eggs, egg whites, milk, cheddar cheese, salt, and pepper to a bowl and beat until well combined.
4. Pour the egg mixture over your chicken mixture evenly and top with Parmesan cheese. Bake for 40 minutes until the top becomes golden brown. Let it cool, and serve!

**Nutritional Info:** Calories: 158; Fat: 8.3g; Carbs: 2.1g; Protein: 17.5g; Fiber: 0.4g

### Spinach Egg Quiche

Time to prepare: 10 minutes
Time to cook: 20 minutes
Servings: 4

**Ingredients:**

- 6 eggs
- ½ cup low-fat milk
- 2 cups fresh baby spinach, chopped
- ¼ cup fresh parsley, chopped
- 1 tablespoon fresh chives, minced
- salt & freshly ground black pepper, to taste

**Directions:**

1. Lightly grease a pie plate and preheat the oven to 400°F.
2. In a bowl, stir together the eggs, milk, salt, and black pepper. Place aside.
3. Combine the spinach and herbs in a separate bowl. After equally distributing this mixture, add the egg mixture over top.
4. Bake for 20 minutes, then let it cool before serving.

**Nutritional Info:** Calories: 120; Fat: 7g; Carbs: 4.3g; Protein: 10.1g; Fiber: 0.98g

## Zucchini & Carrot Quiche

Time to prepare: 10 minutes
Time to cook: 40 minutes
Servings: 3

**Ingredients:**

- 5 eggs
- 1 carrot, peeled and grated
- 1 medium zucchini, peeled, seeded & shredded
- Salt & ground black pepper to taste
- Cooking spray

**Directions:**

1. Preheat your oven to 350°F and spray cooking spray on a small baking dish to gently oil it.
2. Beat the eggs with the salt and black pepper in a large basin. Stir the zucchini and carrots after adding them. Evenly distribute the ingredients in the baking dish you have prepared.
3. Bake for 40 minutes, then serve once it has cooled.

**Nutritional Info:** Calories: 119; Fat: 0.5g; Carbs: 3.9g; Protein: 9.9g; Fiber: 0.9g

## Chicken Spinach Mushroom Quiche

Time to prepare: 10 minutes
Time to cook: 20 minutes
Servings: 4

**Ingredients:**

- 6 eggs
- 1 cup cooked chicken, chopped
- 1 cup fresh baby spinach, chopped
- ½ cup unsweetened almond milk
- ¼ cup fresh mushrooms, sliced
- ¼ cup fresh cilantro, chopped
- 2 tablespoon fresh chives, minced
- Ground black pepper to taste
- Cooking spray

**Directions:**

1. Preheat the oven to 400 degrees Fahrenheit, and lightly spray a pie plate with cooking spray.
2. Combine the eggs, milk, salt, and black pepper in a sizable bowl. Place aside.

3. Place the chicken, herbs, and vegetables in a separate bowl and combine well. Put your chicken mixture in the prepared pie plate's bottom.
4. Evenly distribute the egg mixture over the chicken mixture. Bake for 20 minutes, then let it cool before serving.

**Nutritional Info:** Calories: 158; Fat: 7.1g; Carbs: 2.6g; Protein: 18.2g; Fiber: 0.5g

## Feta Eggs in Tomato Sauce

Time to prepare: 10 minutes
Time to cook: 21 minutes
Servings: 4

**Ingredients:**

- 4 large eggs
- 2 ½ cups tomatoes, seeded & chopped finely
- 3 oz low-fat feta cheese, crumbled
- 1 tablespoon olive oil
- Salt & ground black pepper to taste

**Directions:**

1. In a large cast-iron pan, heat the oil over medium-low heat. Add the tomatoes, stirring frequently, and cook for 4-6 minutes.
2. Using the spoon, spread the mixture into an even layer. Over the tomato mixture, gently crack the eggs, then top with feta cheese and black pepper.
3. Cook the eggs until they are the desired doneness by tightly covering the pan and cooking for 10-15 minutes. Serve warm.

**Nutritional Info:** Calories: 178; Fat: 13.2g; Carbs: 5.6g; Protein: 10.3g; Fiber: 1.3g

## Eggs With Spinach

Time to prepare: 10 minutes
Time to cook: 22 minutes
Servings: 2

**Ingredients:**

- Olive oil cooking spray
- 4 eggs
- 6 cups fresh baby spinach

- 2-3 tablespoon filtered water
- 2-3 tablespoon feta cheese, crumbled
- 2 teaspoon fresh chives, minced
- Ground black pepper to taste

**Directions:**

1. Preheat your oven to 400°F and spray 2 small baking plates with cooking spray to gently oil them.

2. In a large frying pan, add the spinach, water, and salt. Cook for about 3 to 4 minutes, turning occasionally. Completely remove and drain the extra water.

3. Evenly distribute the spinach among the baking dishes. In each baking dish, carefully break two eggs over the spinach. Top equally with feta cheese and a dash of black pepper.

4. Position the baking trays on a large cookie sheet. Bake eggs for 15 to 18 minutes, depending on desired doneness. Remove and serve hot with chives as a garnish.

**Nutritional Info:** Calories: 172; Fat: 11.2g; Carbs: 4.4g; Protein: 15g; Fiber: 1.1g

## Eggs With Beef & Tomatoes

Time to prepare: 10 minutes
Time to cook: 30 minutes
Servings: 4

**Ingredients:**

- 4 eggs
- 12 oz lean ground beef
- 3 cups tomatoes, peeled, seeded & chopped
- 2 oz low-fat feta cheese, crumbled
- 3 tablespoon olive oil
- 2 tablespoon fresh cilantro, chopped
- 2 tablespoon fresh parsley, chopped

**Directions:**

1. Add the cilantro, parsley, salt, and black pepper to your large shallow pan and cook for 2 minutes, stirring frequently, over medium heat.

2. Add the ground beef and simmer, stirring constantly, for approximately 4-5 minutes. Cook for 15 to 20 minutes, stirring now and again after stirring in the tomatoes, salt, and black pepper.

3. Using a spoon, create 4 wells on the surface. Carefully crack an egg into each well, then sprinkle each with a little salt.

4. Cook the egg whites for about 5 minutes, or until they are done to your liking.

5. Take out and sprinkle with the remaining cilantro before serving hot.

**Nutritional Info:** Calories: 361; Fat: 22g; Carbs: 6.2g; Protein: 35.1g; Fiber: 1.7g

## Vanilla Crepes

Time to prepare: 10 minutes
Time to cook: 2 minutes
Servings: 4

**Ingredients:**

- 4 eggs
- 2 cups refined flour
- 2 tablespoon arrowroot powder (if tolerated)
- ½ teaspoon ground cinnamon
- 1 teaspoon vanilla extract
- Olive oil cooking spray

**Directions:**

1. Mix the arrowroot powder, almond flour, and cinnamon in a bowl.

2. In another bowl, beat the eggs plus vanilla extract. Mix both the prepared mixtures until well combined.

3. Lightly grease a large non-stick sauté pan with cooking spray and heat over medium-high heat.

4. Pour enough batter and tilt the pan to spread it in an even layer. Cook for about 1 minute or until the bottom becomes golden brown.

5. Carefully flip the side and cook for about 1 minute more, until golden brown. Repeat with the remaining batter, and serve warm.

**Nutritional Info:** Calories: 107; Fat: 6.3g; Carbs: 5.3g; Protein: 5.6g; Fiber: 0.5g

## Pear Pancakes

Time to prepare: 10 minutes
Time to cook: 15 minutes
Servings: 4
**Ingredients:**

- 2 eggs
- 1 cup pear, peeled mashed
- 1 teaspoon cinnamon
- 2 teaspoon sugar
- 2 cups refined white flour
- 2 teaspoon baking powder
- 2 teaspoon vanilla
- Non-stick cooking spray

**Directions:**

1. In your bowl, beat the eggs until fluffy. Add the baking powder, cinnamon, vanilla, sugar, both flours, and pears, then stir until smooth.
2. Grease your pan using the cooking spray, pour enough batter, and cook until bubbles appear on top.
3. Flip and cook another side until golden. Serve!

**Nutritional Info:** Calories: 174, Fat: 2g, Carbs: 3g, Protein: 5g, Fiber: 2g

## Fluffy Pumpkin Pancakes

Time to prepare: 10 minutes
Time to cook: 4 minutes
Servings: 4
**Ingredients:**

- 2 eggs
- 1 cup refined flour
- 1 tablespoon baking powder
- 1 teaspoon Pumpkin pie spice
- ½ teaspoon salt
- 1 cup pumpkin puree
- ¾ cup + 2 tablespoon low-fat milk
- 3 tablespoon pure maple syrup
- 2 tablespoon olive oil
- 1 teaspoon vanilla extract

**Directions:**

1. In a blender, mix all the ingredients completely. After transferring the mixture to a bowl, wait 10 minutes.
2. Put your nonstick skillet over medium heat and oil it. 14 cups of the mixture should be placed and cooked for approximately 2 minutes on each side. Serve hot.

**Nutritional Info:** Calories: 113; Fat: 4.4g; Carbs: 15.9g; Protein: 3.45g; Fiber: 2g

## Vanilla Maple Pancakes

Time to prepare: 10 minutes
Time to cook: 3 minutes
Servings: 6
**Ingredients:**

- 1 cup refined flour
- 1 cup unsweetened almond milk
- ¼ cup maple syrup
- 2 tablespoon wheat germ
- 1 tablespoon extra-virgin olive oil
- 1 tablespoon baking powder
- 2 teaspoon apple cider vinegar
- 1 teaspoon vanilla extract
- ¼ teaspoon salt

**Directions:**

1. Start by combining the milk and vinegar in a medium bowl. Place aside.
2. In a large basin, combine the flour, wheat germ, baking soda, and salt. Beat until well blended after adding the milk mixture, maple syrup, and vanilla extract.
3. Heat the oil over medium heat in a nonstick wok. Spread the ingredients in a circle at the appropriate thickness. Cook for approximately 1 to 2 minutes before flipping.
4. Carry out step 4 with the leftover mixture. Serve hot.

**Nutritional Info:** Calories: 142; Fat: 3.8g; Carbs: 25.7g; Protein: 3.4g; Fiber: 2.1g

## Ricotta Protein Pancakes

Time to prepare: 10 minutes

Time to cook: 5 minutes
Servings: 4
**Ingredients:**
- 4 eggs
- ½ cup part-skim ricotta cheese
- ¼ cup unsweetened protein powder
- 2 tablespoon olive oil
- ½ teaspoon baking powder
- ½ teaspoon liquid stevia
- Pinch of salt

**Directions:**
1. Add all the ingredients to your blender, excluding the oil, and blend until thoroughly combined.
2. Set the oil in your pan to medium heat. Spread the mixture out evenly after adding the desired quantity.
3. After about 2–3 minutes, flip the food and cook for an additional 1–2 minutes, or until golden brown. The remaining mixture should be used again. Serve hot.

**Nutritional Info:** Calories: 191; Fat: 14g; Carbs: 2.1g; Protein: 14.4g; Fiber: 0g

## Banana Pancakes

Time to prepare: 10 minutes
Time to cook: 5 minutes
Servings: 5
**Ingredients:**
- 2 eggs
- 1 ripe banana, peeled & mashed
- ½ cup unsweetened almond milk
- ¼ cup refined flour
- 1 tablespoon maple syrup
- 2 teaspoon olive oil
- 1 teaspoon apple cider vinegar
- ½ teaspoon ground cinnamon
- ½ teaspoon vanilla extract
- ¼ teaspoon baking powder
- Pinch of salt

**Directions:**
1. In a big bowl, combine the flour, baking powder, cinnamon, and salt.
2. In a different bowl, combine the milk, egg, banana, maple syrup, vinegar, and vanilla.
3. Combine the two components of the prepared mixture thoroughly.
4. Heat the oil over medium heat in your large frying pan. Spread the mixture out evenly after adding the desired quantity.
5. Cook for two to three minutes, then flip and cook for one to two more minutes. The remaining mixture should be used again. Serve hot.

**Nutritional Info:** Calories: 94; Fat: 4.7g; Carbs: 10g; Protein: 3.4g; Fiber: 2g

## Apple Pancakes

Time to prepare: 10 minutes
Time to cook: 4 minutes
Servings: 2
**Ingredients:**
- 1 egg, beaten lightly
- ¼ cup apple, peeled, cored & chopped
- ½ cup unsweetened almond milk
- 1/3 cup refined flour
- 1 tablespoon olive oil
- 1 teaspoon baking powder
- Pinch of salt

**Directions:**
1. Combine the salt, baking powder, and flour in a bowl.
2. In another dish, combine the eggs, almond milk, and olive oil. Just blend the flour mixture with the liquid before adding the apple chunks.
3. Put a nonstick wok that has been oiled over medium heat. Spread the first half of the mixture evenly throughout the area.
4. After around 2–3 minutes, turn the food and cook it for another minute. The leftover mixture should be used again. Serve hot.

**Nutritional Info:** Calories: 181; Fat: 8.7g; Carbs: 14.6g; Protein: 5.4g; Fiber: 2g

## Pumpkin Pancakes

Time to prepare: 15 minutes

Time to cook: 4 minutes

Servings: 4-5

**Ingredients:**

- 2 eggs
- 1 cup pumpkin puree
- 1 cup refined flour
- ¾ cup + 2 tablespoon fat-free milk
- 3 tablespoon maple syrup
- 2 tablespoon olive oil
- 1 tablespoon baking powder
- 1 teaspoon vanilla extract
- ½ teaspoon salt

**Directions:**

1. In a blender, combine all the ingredients completely. After transferring the mixture to a bowl, wait 10 minutes.

2. Put a nonstick wok on medium heat and grease it. Spread out about 14 cups of the mixture in a circular pattern.

3. Cook the remaining mixture for an additional 2 minutes on each side. Serve hot.

**Nutritional Info:** Calories: 113; Fat: 4.4g; Carbs: 16.5g; Protein: 3.6g; Fiber: 2g

## Cheese Tomato Pancake

Time to prepare: 10 minutes

Time to cook: 5 minutes

Servings: 3

**Ingredients:**

- 2 beaten eggs
- 1 canned tomato, peeled & finely chopped
- ½ cup refined flour
- ½ cup cottage cheese, cubed
- 1 teaspoon olive oil
- A pinch of Himalayan salt

**Directions:**

1. In a bowl, mix the tomatoes, cheese, flour, and salt.

2. Add 1/4 cup of the batter to the hot oil in your pan and cook for two to three minutes.

3. Within two minutes, flip and cook the other side. Serve after reusing the leftover batter.

**Nutritional Info:** Calories: 272; Fat: 9.8g; Carbs: 36g; Protein: 16g; Fiber: 1.2g

## Melon And Sweet Potato Cakes

Time to prepare: 10 minutes

Time to cook: 10 minutes

Servings: 2

**Ingredients:**

- 1 cup cooked melon
- 1 cup sweet potato, peeled, diced & cooked
- 2-3 tablespoon white flour
- 2 tablespoon olive oil
- 1 teaspoon old bay seasoning
- ½ teaspoon salt

**Directions:**

1. Fill the dish with everything except the oil. Mix the ingredients to make a fairly sticky dough, then form it into flat circles.

2. In your grill pan, heat the olive oil to medium heat. When the dough is added to the pan, cook it till golden brown for around 4-5 minutes.

3. Cook for 4-5 minutes, then flip. Let it cool before serving.

**Nutritional Info:** Calories: 260; Fat: 7.5g; Carbs: 46g; Protein: 4g; Fiber: 2.6g

## Apple Cider Cinnamon Waffles

Time to prepare: 15 minutes

Time to cook: 10 minutes

Servings: 4

**Ingredients:**

- 1¼ cup unsweetened almond milk
- 1 cup refined flour
- 3 tablespoon water
- 1 tablespoon apple cider vinegar
- 1 tablespoon ground flaxseed
- 1 tablespoon erythritol
- 1¼ teaspoon baking powder

- 1 teaspoon baking soda
- ¼ teaspoon ground cinnamon
- ¼ teaspoon salt

**Directions:**

1. Combine almond milk and vinegar in a bowl. Leave it alone for five minutes.

2. Combine water and ground flaxseed in a dish. Set it aside until it thickens, approximately 5 minutes.

3. In a different bowl, combine the flour, erythritol, cinnamon, baking powder, baking soda, and salt.

4. Pour the milk and vinegar into the flaxseed mixture bowl and stir to combine. Add the flour mixture and blend just enough. Wait for five to ten minutes.

5. Grease the waffle maker and preheat it. Once there is enough batter added, fry for 5 minutes on each side until golden. Serve warm and repeat with the leftover mixture.

**Nutritional Info:** Calories: 125; Fat: 2.6g; Carbs: 23.2g; Protein: 4.4g; Fiber: 2.4g


## Vanilla Egg White Waffles

Time to prepare: 10 minutes
Time to cook: 5 minutes
Servings: 2

**Ingredients:**

- 6 egg whites
- ¼ cup refined white flour
- ¼ cup fat-free milk
- 1 tablespoon pure maple syrup
- 1 teaspoon baking powder
- ¼ teaspoon vanilla extract

**Directions:**

1. Lightly grease the waffle iron while it is warm.

2. In a big bowl, combine the flour and baking powder. Mix well after adding the last of the fixings.

3. Fill the waffle maker with half of the mixture and heat it up. Waffles should be cooked for 3 to 5 minutes or until golden brown.

4. Carry out step 4 with the leftover mixture. Serve hot.

**Nutritional Info:** Calories: 102; Fat: 0.5g; Carbs: 11.2g; Protein: 12.1g; Fiber: 0.7g


## Lemon Cheese Waffles

Time to prepare: 10 minutes
Time to cook: 4 minutes
Servings: 2

**Ingredients:**

- 1 large egg
- ½ cup part-skim mozzarella cheese, shredded
- 2 tablespoon refined white flour
- ¼ teaspoon baking powder
- 1 teaspoon fresh lemon juice
- 2-3 drops of liquid stevia

**Directions:**

1. Grease the tiny waffle iron after preheating it.

2. In a medium bowl, blend all the ingredients well. Put half of the mixture into the waffle iron that has been preheated and cook for around 3–4 minutes.

3. Carry out step 3 with the leftover mixture. Serve hot.

**Nutritional Info:** Calories: 98; Fat: 7.1g; Carbs: 2.2g; Protein: 6.7g; Fiber: 0.8g

Cheesy Pumpkin Waffles

Time to prepare: 10 minutes
Time to cook: 4 minutes
Servings: 2

**Ingredients:**

- 1 egg, beaten
- ½ cup part-skim mozzarella cheese, shredded
- 1 tablespoon canned solid pumpkin
- ¼ teaspoon ground cinnamon

**Directions:**

1. Grease the mini waffle iron after preheating it.

2. Combine all of the ingredients in a

medium bowl.

3. Spoon half of the mixture into a waffle iron that has been preheated and cook for 3 to 4 minutes.

4. Carry out step 4 with the leftover mixture. Serve hot.

**Nutritional Info:** Calories: 56; Fat: 3.5g; Carbs: 1.4g; Protein: 4.9g; Fiber: 0.4g

### Potato Herbed Waffles

Time to prepare: 15 minutes
Time to cook: 8-10 minutes
Servings: 4

**Ingredients:**
- 2 medium potatoes, peeled, grated & squeezed
- 1 teaspoon fresh thyme, minced
- 1 teaspoon fresh rosemary, minced
- Salt & ground black pepper to taste

**Directions:**
1. Grease the tiny waffle iron after preheating it.

2. Combine all the ingredients in a large bowl.

3. Fill the waffle iron with 1/4 of the potato mixture. In 8 to 10 minutes, or until golden brown, cook.

4. Once you've used up all of the mixture, serve.

**Nutritional Info:** Calories: 73; Fat: 0.2g; Carbs: 17.1g; Protein: 1.5g; Fiber: 1.5g

### Cheesy Spinach Waffles

Time to prepare: 10 minutes
Time to cook: 5 minutes
Servings: 4

**Ingredients:**
- 1 large egg, beaten
- 4 oz frozen spinach, thawed & squeezed dry
- 1 cup part-skim ricotta cheese, crumbled
- ½ cup part-skim Mozzarella cheese, shredded
- ¼ cup low-fat Parmesan cheese, grated
- Salt & ground black pepper to taste

**Directions:**
1. Grease the tiny waffle iron after preheating it.

2. In a medium bowl, combine all the cheese, spinach, salt, and black pepper.

3. Spoon 1/4 of the mixture onto a waffle iron that has been prepared, and cook for 4-5 minutes, or until golden brown.

4. Carry out step 4 with the leftover mixture. Serve hot.

**Nutritional Info:** Calories: 138; Fat: 7.1g; Carbs: 4.8g; Protein: 11.7g; Fiber: 0.6g

### Cheesy Zucchini Basil Waffles

Time to prepare: 10 minutes
Time to cook: 5 minutes
Servings: 2

**Ingredients:**
- ½ of small zucchini, peeled, seeded, grated & squeezed
- 1 egg, beaten
- ¼ cup part-skim Mozzarella cheese, shredded
- 2 tablespoon low-fat Parmesan cheese, grated
- ¼ teaspoon dried basil, crushed
- Salt & ground black pepper to taste

**Directions:**
1. Grease the mini waffle iron after preheating it.

2. Combine all of the ingredients in a medium bowl.

3. Spoon half of the mixture into a waffle iron that has been preheated, and cook for about 4-5 minutes.

4. Carry out step 4 with the leftover mixture. Serve hot.

**Nutritional Info:** Calories: 64; Fat: 4.1g; Carbs: 1.3g; Protein: 6.1g; Fiber: 0.3g

## Cheesy Chicken Waffles

Time to prepare: 10 minutes
Time to cook: 5 minutes
Servings: 4

**Ingredients:**
- 4 medium eggs
- 1/3 cup unsweetened almond milk
- ¼ cup cooked chicken, chopped finely
- 2 tablespoon part-skim mozzarella cheese, shredded

**Directions:**
1. Grease the waffle maker after it has warmed up.
2. Combine the almond milk, eggs, and sugar in a medium bowl. Stir in the rest of the fixings to ensure a smooth transition.
3. Pour the desired quantity of batter into the waffle maker that has been heated. Cook for approximately 5 minutes, or until done.
4. Carry out step 4 with the leftover mixture. Serve hot.

**Nutritional Info:** Calories: 91; Fat: 5.7g; Carbs: 1.1g; Protein: 9.3g; Fiber: 0.2g

## Ripe Plantain Bran Muffins

Time to prepare: 10 minutes
Time to cook: 18 minutes
Servings: 12 muffins

**Ingredients:**
- 4 large eggs, lightly beaten
- 2 medium ripe plantains, mashed
- 1 ½ cup refined cereal
- 1 cup refined white flour
- 1 cup of low-fat non-dairy milk
- ¼ cup canola oil
- ½ cup stevia
- 2 teaspoon baking powder
- ½ teaspoon salt

**Directions:**
1. Preheat the oven to 400°F.
2. Place the milk and bran cereal in a bowl and set it aside. Stir in the stevia and plantains after adding the eggs and oil.
3. Combine the flour, baking powder, and salt in a separate bowl. Blend the prepared ingredients well.
4. Evenly distribute the batter into your muffin tins that have been lined with paper and bake for 18 minutes, or until golden brown and firm. Before serving, allow it to cool.

**Nutritional Info:** Calories: 325; Fat: 19g; Carbs: 37g; Protein: 3g; Fiber: 2g

## Tuna Spinach Muffins

Time to prepare: 10 minutes
Time to cook: 30 minutes
Servings: 6

**Ingredients:**
- 2 large eggs
- 1 (7-oz.) can of water-packed tuna, drained
- ¼ cup spinach, chopped finely
- 3 oz low-fat cheddar cheese, shredded
- ½ cup low-fat mayonnaise
- 1 tablespoon fresh parsley, chopped
- Salt & ground black pepper to taste

**Directions:**
1. Warm your oven to 350ºF, and grease 6 cups of a muffin tin.
2. In your bowl, add all the ingredients and mix until well combined. Pour the batter into your muffin cups evenly.
3. Bake for 25–30 minutes, until the top becomes golden brown. Let it cool, and serve!

**Nutritional Info:** Calories: 99; Fat: 1.9g; Carbs: 3.4g; Protein: 15.2g; Fiber: 0.1g

## Chicken Egg Muffins

Time to prepare: 15 minutes
Time to cook: 20 minutes
Servings: 8 muffins

**Ingredients:**

- 8 eggs
- 2 tablespoon water
- 8 oz cooked chicken, chopped finely
- Ground black pepper to taste

**Directions:**

1. Warm your oven to 350oF and grease 8 muffin tins.

2. In a bowl, beat the eggs, salt, black pepper, and water until well combined. Add the chicken and stir to combine.

3. Transfer the mixture into the muffin cups evenly. Bake for 18–20 minutes, until golden brown. Let it cool, and serve!

**Nutritional Info:** Calories: 116; Fat: 5.3g; Carbs: 2.7g; Protein: 14.1g; Fiber: 0.4g

## Chicken & Zucchini Muffins

Time to prepare: 10 minutes
Time to cook: 15 minutes
Servings: 8 muffins

**Ingredients:**

- 4 eggs
- ¾ cup cooked chicken, shredded
- ¾ cup zucchini, grate
- 1/3 cup refined flour
- ½ cup low-fat Parmesan cheese, shredded
- ¼ cup low-fat cheddar cheese, grated
- ¼ cup olive oil
- ¼ cup water
- 1 tablespoon fresh oregano, minced
- 1 tablespoon fresh thyme, minced
- ½ teaspoon baking powder
- ¼ teaspoon salt

**Directions:**

1. Preheat your oven to 400 degrees Fahrenheit, and lightly grease an 8-cup muffin tin.

2. In a bowl, combine the eggs, oil, and water and whisk until well combined. Mix well after adding the flour, baking powder, and salt. Mix in the remaining ingredients just until combined.

3. Evenly distribute the muffin batter into the prepared muffin cups. Bake for 13 to 15 minutes, or until golden brown on top. Let it cool before serving.

**Nutritional Info:** Calories: 164; Fat: 12.6g; Carbs: 4.3g; Protein: 9.9g; Fiber: 1.9g

## Chicken Spinach Muffins

Time to prepare: 15 minutes
Time to cook: 45 minutes
Servings: 8

**Ingredients:**

- 8 eggs
- 7 oz cooked chicken, chopped finely
- 1 ½ cup fresh spinach, chopped
- 2 tablespoon filtered water
- 2 tablespoon fresh parsley, chopped finely
- Salt & freshly ground black pepper to taste

**Directions:**

1. Grease a muffin tin with 8 cups and preheat the oven to 350°F.

2. In a bowl, stir together the eggs, water, salt, and black pepper. Stir in the chicken, spinach, and parsley after adding them.

3. Evenly distribute the mixture into the prepared muffin cups. Golden brown will come after 18 to 20 minutes of baking. Let it cool before serving.

**Nutritional Info:** Calories: 103; Fat: 6.6g; Carbs: 1.5g; Protein: 8.9g; Fiber: 0.5g

## Breakfast Bran Muffins

Time to prepare: 10 minutes
Time to cook: 20 minutes
Servings: 10

**Ingredients:**

- 2 eggs
- 2 ½ cups refined white flour
- 2 cups refined cereal

- ½ -quart buttermilk
- 1 cup boiling water
- ½ cup stevia
- ½ cup olive oil
- 2 ½ teaspoon baking soda
- ½ teaspoon salt

**Directions:**

1. Set the oven to 400 degrees.
2. Set aside 1 cup of cereal that has been soaked in 1 cup of boiling water.
3. In a mixer, combine the butter and stevia until well combined. After adding each egg one at a time, beat until fluffy.Add the buttermilk and cereal mixture that has been soaked.
4. Combine the flour, salt, and baking soda in a separate bowl. Don't over-mix the batter as you add the flour mixture.
5. Add the last cup of cereal and stir well. The batter should be evenly distributed among the 10 greased or paper-lined muffin tins.
6. After baking for 15 to 20 minutes, let the dish cool before serving.

**Nutritional Info:** Calories: 440; Fat: 20g; Carbs: 57g; Protein: 9g; Fiber: 3g

## Classic Zucchini Bread

Time to prepare: 20 minutes
Time to cook: 45-50 minutes
Servings: 24 slices

**Ingredients:**

- 3 eggs, beaten
- 3 cup refined white flour
- 2 cups zucchini, peeled, seeded, & grated
- 2 cups Splenda
- 1 cup olive oil
- 2 teaspoon baking soda
- 2 teaspoon vanilla extract
- 1 teaspoon ground cinnamon
- 1 teaspoon ground nutmeg

**Directions:**

1. Preheat the oven to 325°F, place a rack in the middle, and oil two loaf pans.
2. In a large bowl, combine the spices, baking soda, and flour.
3. Add the oil and Splenda to a different big dish and mix well. Beat in the eggs and vanilla extract after adding them.
4. Add the flour mixture and blend just enough. Fold the zucchini in gently.
5. Distribute the ingredients equally among the bread loaf pans. Bake for 45 to 50 minutes, then let it cool before serving.

**Nutritional Info:** Calories: 208; Fat: 10.2g; Carbs: 27.8g; Protein: 2.4g; Fiber: 0.6g

## Carrot Bread

Time to prepare: 15 minutes
Time to cook: 60 minutes
Servings: 10 slices

**Ingredients:**

- 3 eggs
- 3 cups carrot, peeled & grated
- 2 cups refined flour
- 2 tablespoon olive oil
- 1 tablespoon apple cider vinegar
- 1 teaspoon baking powder
- ¼ teaspoon salt

**Directions:**

1. Preheat your oven to 350 degrees Fahrenheit, then line a loaf pan with parchment paper.
2. In a large bowl, combine the flour, baking soda, and salt.
3. In a separate bowl, thoroughly mix the eggs, oil, and vinegar. This mixture should be added and thoroughly combined with the flour mixture. Toss the carrots in.
4. Evenly distribute the mixture into the prepared loaf pan. Bake for an hour, then let it cool before serving.

**Nutritional Info:** Calories: 89; Fat: 6.9g; Carbs: 4.8g; Protein: 3.1g; Fiber: 1.4g

## Apple Oatmeal

Time to prepare: 10 minutes
Time to cook: 1-2 minutes
Servings: 1
**Ingredients:**
- ½ cup instant oatmeal
- ¾ cup water
- ½ cup apples, peeled and cooked pureed
- 1 teaspoon maple syrup

**Directions:**
1. Combine the oats, water, and apples in a bowl that can be microwaved. Within one to two minutes, cook on high in the microwave.
2. Cook for another 30 seconds after thoroughly stirring. Add some maple syrup, and then serve.

**Nutritional Info:** Calories: 295; Fat: 7g; Carbs: 47g; Protein: 13g; Fiber: 5g

## Spiced Oatmeal

Time to prepare: 2 minutes
Time to cook: 2 minutes
Servings: 2
**Ingredients:**
- 1 cup quick oats
- 1 cup water
- 1 tablespoon almond butter
- ¼ teaspoon ground ginger
- ¼ teaspoon ground cinnamon
- A dash of ground nutmeg
- A dash of ground clove

**Directions:**
1. In a bowl that can be heated in the microwave, combine the oats and water. Stir well after 45 seconds in the microwave, then cook for an additional 30 to 45 seconds.
2. Before serving, add the spices and drizzle the almond butter.

**Nutritional Info:** Calories: 467; Fat: 11g; Carbs: 33g; Protein: 6g; Fiber: 4g

## Peanut Butter Banana Oatmeal

Time to prepare: 5 minutes
Time to cook: 0 minutes
Servings: 1
**Ingredients:**
- 1 cup quick oats
- ½ sliced banana
- 1 tablespoon peanut butter, unsweetened
- ¼ teaspoon cinnamon (optional)

**Directions:**
1. Combine all the ingredients in a dish, cover it, and refrigerate overnight before serving.

**Nutritional Info:** Calories: 645; Fat: 32g; Carbs: 65g, Protein: 26g; Fiber: 5g

## Peach Banana Oatmeal

Time to prepare: 10 minutes
Time to cook: 0 minutes
Servings: 2
**Ingredients:**
- 1 medium banana, peeled and chopped
- ½ cup quick-cooking oats
- ½ cup peach, peeled & diced
- ½ cup plain nonfat Greek yogurt
- 2/3 cup skim milk
- 1 tablespoon chia seeds
- ½ teaspoon vanilla

**Directions:**
1. In a dish with a cover, combine the oats, milk, yogurt, chia seeds, and vanilla. 12 hours should be spent cooling.
2. Before serving, add the fruits on top.

**Nutritional Info:** Calories: 282; Fat: 6g; Carbs: 48g; Protein: 10g; Fiber: 2g

## Coconut Chia Seed Pudding

Time to prepare: 5 minutes + chilling time
Time to cook: 0 minutes

Servings: 2

**Ingredients:**

- 6 tablespoon chia seeds
- 2 cups unsweetened coconut milk

**Directions:**

1. Combine all the ingredients in a bowl, cover it, and refrigerate overnight before using.

**Nutritional Info:** Calories: 223; Fat: 12g, Carbs: 18g; Protein: 10g; Fiber: 2g

## Strawberry Cashew Chia Pudding

Time to prepare: 10 minutes
Time to cook: 0 minutes
Servings: 2

**Ingredients:**

- 6 tablespoon chia seeds
- 2 cups unsweetened cashew milk,
- Strawberries, for topping

**Directions:**

1. In a dish, combine the chia seeds and milk. Cover and refrigerate for at least eight hours.
2. Before serving, stir in the berries.

**Nutritional Info:** Calories: 223; Fat: 12g; Carbs: 18g; Protein: 10g; Fiber: 2g

## Breakfast Hash with Sausage & Spinach

Time to prepare: 10 minutes
Time to cook: 15 minutes
Servings: 4

**Ingredients:**

- 1 lb. ground turkey sausage
- 4 small peeled & chopped sweet potatoes
- 2 apples, cored and chopped
- 1 garlic clove, minced
- 10 oz chopped spinach
- Salt & pepper to taste

**Directions:**

1. In the pan, brown the sausage until no pink is visible.
2. Once the spinach and apples are cooked, add the additional ingredients and simmer. Serve hot with appropriate seasoning.

**Nutritional Info:** Calories: 544; Fat: 2g; Carbs: 65g; Protein: 11g; Fiber: 2g

## Potato Hash with Egg Scramble

Time to prepare: 10 minutes
Time to cook: 25 minutes
Servings: 2

**Ingredients:**

- 2 eggs, beaten
- 1/2 chopped onion
- 2 cups potatoes, peeled & cubed
- 2 tablespoon extra-virgin olive oil
- 1/2 teaspoon sea salt
- A pinch of freshly ground black pepper

**Directions:**

1. In your large nonstick pan, heat the olive oil over medium-high heat.
2. Include the sweet potato and onion. Add salt and black pepper, stir frequently, and cook the potatoes until they are tender and browned.
3. Place your dishes with the potatoes.
4. Lower the heat to medium-low and add the remaining olive oil, stirring. Add the eggs, cook for three to four minutes, and season to taste.
5. Place the egg on top of the potato mixture, then serve!

**Nutritional Info:** Calories: 320; Fat: 19g; Carbs: 30.3g; Protein: 9.1g; Fiber: 4g

## Melon Carrot Protein Porridge

Time to prepare: 10 minutes
Time to cook: 8 minutes
Servings: 2

**Ingredients:**

- 1 cup cantaloupe or honeydew melon, peeled & grated
- 1 small carrot, peeled & grated
- 1 cup milk
- 1 tablespoon white flour
- 1 teaspoon olive oil
- 2 tablespoon organic honey
- 1 teaspoon whey protein powder

**Directions:**

1. In a saucepan over low heat, warm the olive oil. Cook the carrots and melon for two to three minutes.

2. After adding the milk and honey, simmer the mixture for an additional 5 minutes over medium heat while stirring constantly.

3. Mix together a portion of the hot milk and the white flour, then add to the mixture. Cook until a little thickening occurs.

4. Put the prepared dish in a bowl, top with extra honey, and serve it with canned fruit (optional).

**Nutritional Info:** Calories: 317; Fat: 6.8g; Carbs: 51g; Protein: 10.9g; Fiber: 1.7g

## Breakfast Maple Cornflakes

Time to prepare: 10 minutes
Time to cook: 20 minutes
Servings: 2

**Ingredients:**

- 2 eggs, lightly beaten
- 2 cups nondairy milk
- 1½ cups crushed corn flakes
- 2-4 tablespoon maple syrup
- 1 tablespoon olive oil
- 1 teaspoon whey protein
- A pinch of salt & cinnamon

**Directions:**

1. Grease a baking pan and preheat your oven to 350 degrees Fahrenheit.

2. In a bowl, combine all the dry ingredients, then spread them out on the pan.

3. Add the milk and beaten eggs to the pan and bake for 20 minutes. Serve warm or cold, and if desired, top with canned fruit.

**Nutritional Info:** Calories: 328; Fat: 10.2g; Carbs: 42.4g; Protein: 16.2g; Fiber: 0.7g

## Pear And Cornflakes Granola

Time to prepare: 15 minutes
Time to cook: 25 minutes
Servings: 2

**Ingredients:**

- 1 pear, grated largely
- 2 cups cornflakes
- 1 teaspoon stevia
- 2 teaspoon olive oil

**Directions:**

1. Grease a baking sheet and preheat the oven to 350°F.

2. Combine the pears and cornflakes in a bowl.

3. Melt the sugar and olive oil together in your saucepan. Stir the two ingredients well together to coat.

4. Spread this mixture out on your baking sheet and bake for 25 minutes, stirring every 10 minutes, until golden brown. Let it cool before serving.

**Nutritional Info:** Calories: 185; Fat: 6.1g; Carbs: 33.6g; Protein: 2g; Fiber: 2.1g

## Chicken Lettuce Wraps

Time to prepare: 15 minutes
Time to cook: 10 minutes
Servings: 5
**Ingredients:**
For Chicken:
- 1¼ lb. ground chicken
- 1 teaspoon fresh ginger, minced
- 2 tablespoon olive oil
- Salt & freshly ground black pepper to taste

For Wraps:
- 10 romaine lettuce leaves
- 1½ cup carrot, peeled & julienned
- 2 tablespoon fresh parsley, chopped finely
- 2 tablespoon fresh lime juice

**Directions:**
1. In a pan set over medium heat, add the oil and ginger; cook for approximately a minute.
2. After adding the ground chicken, salt, and black pepper, simmer for 7-9 minutes while breaking up the meat with a wooden spoon. Take the food off the stove and let it cool.
3. Distribute the lettuce leaves among the dishes. Over each lettuce leaf, arrange the cooked chicken and garnish with cilantro and carrot. Serve right after adding lime juice.

**Nutritional Info:** Calories: 240; Fat: 15.1g; Carbs: 6.2g; Protein: 20.9g; Fiber: 2.34g

## Mushroom Curry

Time to prepare: 15 minutes
Time to cook: 18 minutes
Servings: 6
**Ingredients:**
- 5 cups fresh button mushrooms, sliced
- 2 cups fresh shiitake mushrooms, sliced
- 2 cups tomatoes, peeled, seeded & chopped
- 1½ cup water
- ¼ cup fat-free plain yogurt, whipped
- 2 tablespoon olive oil
- 1 teaspoon fresh ginger, chopped
- ¼ teaspoon ground turmeric
- Salt & ground black pepper to taste

**Directions:**
1. In a food processor, blend the tomatoes with 1/4 cup of water until a homogeneous puree forms.
2. Saute the ginger and turmeric in a skillet with the oil over medium heat for approximately a minute. Cook for approximately 5 minutes after incorporating the tomato paste.
3. Add the yogurt, mushrooms, and remaining water. Bring to a boil. Cook for around 10 to 12 minutes, stirring now and again.
4. Add salt and black pepper to taste and serve hot.

**Nutritional Info:** Calories: 70; Fat: 5g; Carbs: 5.3g; Protein: 3g; Fiber: 1.4g

## Beef Skewers

Time to prepare: 10 minutes
Time to cook: 12 minutes
Servings: 5
**Ingredients:**
- 1½ lb. beef tenderloin, trimmed & cut into 1-inch cubes
- 2 tablespoon extra-virgin olive oil
- 2 tablespoon fresh lemon juice
- 1 tablespoon fresh thyme, chopped
- 1 tablespoon fresh oregano, chopped
- 1 teaspoon lemon zest, grated

- Salt & ground black pepper to taste

**Directions:**

1. 1. In a large bowl, combine all the ingredients—except the beef cubes—and stir until well combined. Add the beef cubes and generously cover with the mixture.

   2. To marinate for the entire night, cover, and chill.

   3. Grease the grill grate and heat up the outdoor grill to medium-high heat.

2. 4. Thread the pre-soaked bamboo skewers with beef cubes. The skewers should be placed on the grill and cooked for 10 to 12 minutes, flipping every two to three minutes. Serve right away.

**Nutritional Info:** Calories: 279; Fat: 5.2g; Carbs: 1g; Protein: 33g; Fiber: 0.2g

### Roasted Pumpkin Curry

Time to prepare: 15 minutes
Time to cook: 38 minutes
Servings: 4

**Ingredients:**

For Roasted Pumpkin:
- 1 medium sugar pumpkin, peeled & cubed
- 1 teaspoon olive oil
- Salt to taste

For Curry:
- 2 large tomatoes, peeled, seeded & chopped
- 2 cups homemade vegetable broth
- 2 tablespoon fresh parsley, chopped
- 1 tablespoon fresh lime juice
- 1 teaspoon olive oil
- Salt & ground black pepper to taste

**Directions:**

1. Preheat your oven to 400 degrees Fahrenheit and cover a large baking sheet with parchment paper.
2. Place all of the prepared roasted pumpkin ingredients in a large bowl and mix to combine. Put the pumpkin mixture in a single layer on the baking sheet that has been prepared.
3. Roast for 20 to 25 minutes, turning once at the halfway point.
4. In the meanwhile, sauté the tomatoes for two to three minutes in the oil in your big pan over medium-high heat.
5. Bring to a boil the broth, salt, and black pepper. Set the heat to low and simmer for ten minutes.
6. Add the parsley and roasted pumpkin, and cook for an additional 10 minutes. Serve warm.

**Nutritional Info:** Calories: 76; Fat: 3.2g; Carbs: 9g; Protein: 2.1g; Fiber: 3.9g

### Cheesy Basil Chicken Skewers

Time to prepare: 15 minutes + marinating time
Time to cook: 7 minutes
Servings: 4

**Ingredients:**

- 1¼ lb. chicken breast, boneless & skinless, sliced into 1-inch cubes
- 1 cup fresh basil leaves, chopped
- ¼ cup low-fat Parmesan cheese, grated
- 3 tablespoon olive oil
- Salt & freshly ground black pepper to taste

**Directions:**

1. In a food processor, blend the cheese, oil, basil, garlic, salt, and black pepper until smooth. Place it in a sizable bowl.
2. Stir in the chicken cubes thoroughly. Marinate for 4-5 hours, covered and chilled.
3. Grease the grill grate and heat the grill

to a medium-high temperature. Threaded chicken cubes onto previously soaked wooden skewers

4. After putting the skewers on the grill, cook them for 3 to 4 minutes. Cook for another 2 to 3 minutes after flipping.

5. Remove and set aside on a platter for about five minutes prior to serving. Serve warm.

**Nutritional Info:** Calories: 282; Fat: 15.7g; Carbs: 0.4g; Protein: 33.3g; Fiber: 0.1g

## Shrimp Maple Skewers

Time to prepare: 15 minutes
Time to cook: 8 minutes
Servings: 4
**Ingredients:**
- 1 lb. medium raw shrimp, peeled & deveined
- ¼ cup olive oil
- 2 tablespoon fresh lime juice
- 1 teaspoon maple syrup
- ¼ teaspoon ground cumin
- Salt & ground black pepper to taste

**Directions:**
1. Combine all the ingredients in a large bowl, except the shrimp. Add the shrimp and thoroughly sprinkle it with the herb mixture. Within 30 minutes, marinate in the refrigerator.

2. Grease the grill grate and heat the grill to a medium-high temperature. Shrimp are threaded onto wooden skewers that have been pre-soaked.

3. After putting the skewers on the grill, roast them for 2-4 minutes on each side. Remove and set aside for about five minutes before serving.

**Nutritional Info:** Calories: 211; Fat: 15.2g; Carbs: 2.5g; Protein: 16g; Fiber: 0.7g

## Pan-Seared Scallops

Time to prepare: 10 minutes
Time to cook: 7 minutes
Servings: 4
**Ingredients:**
- 1¼ lb. fresh sea scallops, side muscles removed
- 2 tablespoon olive oil
- 1 tablespoon fresh parsley, minced
- Salt & ground black pepper to taste

**Directions:**
1. Season the scallops with black pepper and salt.

2. In a large skillet, heat the oil over medium-high heat. Cook the scallops for two to three minutes on each side.

3. Add the parsley, remove, and then hot-serve.

**Nutritional Info:** Calories: 161; Fat: 7.8g; Carbs: 4.7g; Protein: 17.1g; Fiber: 0g

## Shrimp Tomato Salad

Time to prepare: 10 minutes
Time to cook: 3 minutes
Servings: 5
**Ingredients:**
- 1 lb. shrimp, peeled and deveined
- 3 tomatoes, peeled, seeded, and sliced
- 1 lemon, quartered
- ¼ cup olives pitted
- ¼ cup fresh cilantro, chopped finely
- 2 tablespoon olive oil
- 2 teaspoon fresh lemon juice
- Salt & ground black pepper to taste

**Directions:**
1. Put the quartered lemon and a little salt in a skillet and heat it until it boils. After adding the shrimp, simmer for 2 to 3 minutes, or until pink and opaque.

2. Using a slotted spoon, place the shrimp in a large dish of cold water to halt the frying. Completely drain the shrimp, then pat it dry with paper towels.

3. In a small bowl, add the oil, lemon juice, salt, and black pepper. Beat well to blend.
4. Arrange the cilantro, shrimp, tomato, olives, and cheese on serving dishes. Serve after drizzling with the oil mixture.
**Nutritional Info:** Calories: 136; Fat: 7.6g; Carbs: 3.9g; Protein: 13.4g; Fiber: 1.7g

### Tomato Salmon Bowl

Time to prepare: 10 minutes
Time to cook: 0 minutes
Servings: 2
**Ingredients:**
- 6 oz. cooked salmon, chopped
- ¼ cup tomato, peeled, seeded, and chopped
- ¼ cup low-fat mozzarella cheese, cubed
- 1 tablespoon fresh dill, chopped
- 1 teaspoon fresh lemon juice
- Salt, to taste

**Directions:**
1. Place all the ingredients in a medium bowl and mix to incorporate.
2. Serve right away.
**Nutritional Info:** Calories: 186; Fat: 11.3g; Carbs: 1.1g; Protein: 20g; Fiber: 0.2g

### Ground Chicken with Tomatoes

Time to prepare: 10 minutes
Time to cook: 13 minutes
Servings: 4
**Ingredients:**
- 1¼ lb. ground chicken
- 2 tomatoes, peeled, seeded & chopped
- 2 tablespoon olive oil
- 2 tablespoon fresh parsley, chopped
- Salt & ground black pepper to taste

**Directions:**
1. Heat the oil in your pan over medium heat, then cook the ground chicken for 6 to 8 minutes.
2. Add the tomatoes and cook, stirring frequently, for about 4-5 minutes. Serve hot after adding parsley, salt, and black pepper.
**Nutritional Info:** Calories: 274; Fat: 18.6g; Carbs: 2.6g; Protein: 25.3g; Fiber: 0.8g

### Beet Pasta with Spinach

Time to prepare: 10 minutes
Time to cook: 14 minutes
Servings: 2
**Ingredients:**
- 2 medium beets, trimmed, peeled & spiralized
- 2 cups fresh spinach, chopped
- 2 tablespoon olive oil, divided
- Salt & ground black pepper to taste

**Directions:**
1. Preheat your oven to 425 degrees Fahrenheit and lightly grease a sizable baking sheet.
2. Spread the prepared baking sheet with the beet pasta. Sprinkle with salt and black pepper, drizzle with 1 tablespoon of oil, and then gently toss to coat.
3. Roast for 5 to 10 minutes, depending on the desired level of doneness.
4. In the meantime, cook the spinach in the remaining oil in a small pan over medium heat for 3 to 4 minutes. After adding salt and black pepper, turn off the heat.
5. Place the pasta and spinach in a sizable bowl and combine thoroughly. Serve right away.
**Nutritional Info:** Calories: 171; Fat: 14.g; Carbs: 11.1g; Protein: 2.5g; Fiber: 2.6g

### Potatoes With Tomatoes

Time to prepare: 10 minutes
Time to cook: 35 minutes
Servings: 6
**Ingredients:**

- 1½ lb. Yukon Gold potatoes, peeled & cubed
- 3 cups tomatoes, peeled, seeded & chopped
- 1 cup water
- 2 tablespoon fresh lime juice
- 2 tablespoon olive oil
- Salt & ground black pepper to taste

**Directions:**

1. In your large skillet, heat the oil over medium heat. Cook the potatoes and tomatoes for about 4–5 minutes.

2. Add the water, cover, and simmer for 20 to 30 minutes. Remove from the heat after adding the lime juice, salt, and black pepper. Serve warm.

**Nutritional Info:** Calories: 89; Fat: 4.9g; Carbs: 11.2g; Protein: 1.7g; Fiber: 1.7g

## Shrimp, Sausage, and Veggie Skillet

Time to prepare: 15 minutes
Time to cook: 13 minutes
Servings: 3

**Ingredients:**

- 1 lb. shrimp, peeled and deveined
- 6 oz cooked turkey sausage, chopped
- 1 zucchini, chopped
- 2 garlic cloves, minced
- 1/2 medium yellow onion, chopped
- 1/4 cup chicken broth
- 3 tablespoon organic olive oil, divided
- Salt & freshly ground black pepper to taste

**Directions:**

1. In a large skillet, heat 1 tablespoon of oil over medium-high heat. After about 3–4 minutes, add the shrimp and then transfer it to a bowl.

2. Heat the remaining oil in the same skillet at medium heat. For approximately 4 minutes, add the onion and continue to sauté.

3. Add the meat and zucchini, then

simmer for about two minutes. Cook the shrimp and garlic together for about a minute.

4. Add the broth and stir well. Black pepper and salt should be added before cooking for about a minute. Serve warm.

**Nutritional Info:** Calories: 430; Fat: 30.9g; Carbs: 7.6g; Protein: 29.5g; Fiber: 2.6g

## Beef & Veggie Burgers

Time to prepare: 15 minutes
Time to cook: 12 minutes
Servings: 8

**Ingredients:**

- 1 carrot, peeled & chopped finely
- 1 large beet, trimmed, peeled & chopped finely
- 1 lb. lean ground beef
- 3 tablespoon olive oil
- 1 tablespoon fresh cilantro, chopped finely
- Salt & ground black pepper to taste

**Directions:**

1. To your large bowl, add all the ingredients (except the oil) and stir to thoroughly combine. From the mixture, form 8 patties of the same size.

2. Prepare the patties in two batches and cook them for 4-6 minutes per side in a large nonstick sauté pan with the olive oil heated to medium heat. Serve warm.

**Nutritional Info:** Calories: 159; Fat: 8.8g; Carbs: 2g; Protein: 17.5g; Fiber: 0.4g

## Sea Scallops with Spinach and Bacon

Time to prepare: 10 minutes
Time to cook: 21 minutes
Servings: 4

**Ingredients:**

- 1 ½ lb. jumbo sea scallops
- 3 turkey bacon slices

- 12 oz fresh baby spinach
- 1 cup onion, chopped
- 6 garlic cloves, minced
- Salt & freshly ground black pepper to taste

**Directions:**

1. Preheat a sizable nonstick skillet over high heat. Cook the bacon for 8–10 minutes after adding it.
2. Empty the skillet of all but 1 tablespoon of bacon fat, then transfer the bacon to a bowl. Bacon should be chopped and set aside.
3. Add salt and black pepper to the skillet before adding the scallops. Cook for approximately 5 minutes on high heat, turning once every 2 1/2 minutes.
4. Insert the scallops in a different bowl. To keep them warm, cover them with foil paper.
5. Add the onion and garlic to the same skillet. Set the heat to medium-high and sauté the vegetables for about 3 minutes.
6. Add the spinach and cook for two to three minutes. Add salt and black pepper to taste. Get rid of the heat.
7. Distribute the spinach between serving trays. Add scallops and bacon evenly on top. Serve right away.

**Nutritional Info:** Calories: 241; Fat: 8.5g; Carbs: 13.5g; Protein: 27.8 g; Fiber: 2.6 g

### Liver with Onion and Parsley

Time to prepare: 15 minutes
Time to cook: 22 minutes
Servings: 4

**Ingredients:**

- 1 lb. grass-fed beef liver, cut into 1/2-inch-thick slices
- 1/2 cup fresh parsley
- 3 tablespoon olive oil, divided
- 2 large onions, sliced
- 2 tablespoon freshly squeezed lemon juice

- Salt & ground black pepper to taste

**Directions:**

1. Heat 1 tablespoon of oil in a large skillet over high heat. Saute for around five minutes after adding the salt and onions. Sauté for an additional 10-15 minutes after adjusting to medium heat. Place aside.
2. Add one more tablespoon of oil to the same skillet and bring to a medium-high heat. Black pepper and salt should be added, along with the liver. Cook until browned for about 1-2 minutes.
3. Turn over and cook for about 1-2 minutes, or until browned. Place aside.
4. Set the remaining oil in the skillet to medium heat. Stir well after adding the cooked onion, parsley, and lemon juice. For two to three minutes, cook.
5. Arrange the onion mixture on top of the liver, then serve right away.

**Nutritional Info:** Calories: 274; Fat: 14g; Carbs: 11.8g; Protein: 24g; Fiber: 1.4 g

### Egg & Avocado Endive Wraps

Time to prepare: 20 minutes
Time to cook: 0 minutes
Servings: 5

**Ingredients:**

- 4 organic hard-boiled eggs, peeled & finely chopped
- 4-5 endive bulbs
- 2 cooked turkey bacon slices, chopped
- 1 ripe avocado, peeled, pitted, & chopped
- 1 tablespoon freshly squeezed lemon juice
- 1 tablespoon fresh parsley, chopped
- 2 tablespoon celery stalk, chopped
- Salt & freshly ground black pepper to taste

**Directions:**

1. In a bowl, combine the avocado with the lemon juice and mash until smooth.

Eggs, celery, parsley, salt, and black pepper should also be added. Blend well.
2. Split the endive leaves, then evenly distribute the avocado mixture over them. Serve right away and top with bacon.
**Nutritional Info:** Calories: 183; Fat: 11.1g; Carbs: 12.7g; Protein: 10.9g; Fiber: 1g

## Greek Cucumber Salad

Time to prepare: 10 minutes
Time to cook: 0 minutes
Servings: 4
**Ingredients:**
- 4 medium cucumbers, peeled, seeded, & chopped
- ½ cup nonfat Greek yogurt
- 1½ tablespoon fresh dill, chopped
- 1 tablespoon fresh lemon juice
- Salt & freshly ground black pepper to taste

**Directions:**
1. Mix all the ingredients well in a big bowl.
2. 2. Serve right away.

**Nutritional Info:** Calories: 54; Fat: 0.8g; Carbs: 8.6g; Protein: 4.5g; Fiber: 1g

## Beef & Spinach Burgers

Time to prepare: 15 minutes
Time to cook: 12 minutes
Servings: 4
**Ingredients:**
- 1 egg, beaten
- 1 lb. lean ground beef
- 1 cup fresh baby spinach leaves, chopped
- ½ cup sun-dried tomatoes, peeled, seeded, and chopped
- ¼ cup low-fat feta cheese, crumbled
- 2 tablespoon olive oil
- Salt & ground black pepper to taste

**Directions:**

1. To a large bowl, add all the ingredients (excluding the oil) and stir to thoroughly blend. The ingredients should be divided into four equal patties.
2. In a cast-iron pan, heat the oil over medium-high heat. When the patties are done, fry them for approximately 5 to 6 minutes on each side. Serve right away.
**Nutritional Info:** Calories: 259; Fat: 17.1g; Carbs: 1.5g; Protein: 25.6g; Fiber: 0.7g

## Cucumber Tomato Salad

Time to prepare: 10 minutes
Time to cook: 0 minutes
Servings: 5
**Ingredients:**
- 2 cups cucumbers, peeled, seeded, & chopped
- 2 cups red tomatoes, peeled, seeded, & chopped
- 2 tablespoon extra-virgin olive oil
- 2 tablespoon fresh lime juice
- Salt, to taste

**Directions:**
1. Combine all the ingredients in a large serving dish and toss to evenly coat.
2. Serve right away.
**Nutritional Info:** Calories: 72; Fat: 5.9g; Carbs: 5.1g; Protein: 0.9g; Fiber: 1.1g

## European Beet Soup

Time to prepare: 10 minutes
Time to cook: 5 minutes
Servings: 3
**Ingredients:**
- 2 cups beets, trimmed, peeled, & chopped
- 2 cups fat-free yogurt
- 4 teaspoon fresh lemon juice
- 2 tablespoon fresh dill
- 1 tablespoon fresh chives, minced
- Salt to taste

**Directions:**

1. Pulse all the ingredients, save the chives, in a high-speed blender until they are well combined.
2. Place the soup in a pan over medium heat, and heat it up for approximately 3 minutes.
3. Immediately serve with chives as a garnish.

**Nutritional Info:** Calories: 122; Fat: 0.2g; Carbs: 14.6g; Protein: 16g; Fiber: 2.6g

## Pasta with Asparagus

Time to prepare: 10 minutes
Time to cook: 10 minutes
Servings: 4

**Ingredients:**

- 1 lb. asparagus, trimmed & cut into 1½-inch pieces
- ½ lb. cooked hot pasta, drained
- 2 tablespoon olive oil
- Salt & freshly ground black pepper to taste

**Directions:**

1. In a large cast-iron pan over medium heat, heat the oil. Add the asparagus, salt, and pepper, and cook for 8 to 10 minutes, tossing periodically.
2. Add the heated pasta and toss to thoroughly coat. Serve right away.

**Nutritional Info:** Calories: 171; Fat: 7.7g; Carbs: 21.1g; Protein: 5.3g; Fiber: 2.9g

## Versatile Mac' n Cheese

Time to prepare: 15 minutes
Time to cook: 8-9 minutes
Servings: 3

**Ingredients:**

- 2 cups refined elbow macaroni, cooked & drained

- 1½ lb. butternut squash, peeled, cubed
- 1 cup low-fat Swiss cheese, shredded
- 1/3 cup low-fat milk
- 1 tablespoon olive oil
- Salt & freshly ground black pepper to taste

**Directions:**

1. Boil the squash cubes for approximately 6 minutes, or until they are tender. Completely drain the squash cubes, then add them back to the pan.
2. Mash the squash with a fork and cook it over low heat. Cook for approximately 2–3 minutes while stirring continually, adding the cheese and milk.
3. Include the macaroni and whisk in the oil, salt, and black pepper. Serve immediately after removing from the heat.

**Nutritional Info:** Calories: 322; Fat: 7.7g; Carbs: 44.6g; Protein: 17.3g; Fiber: 1.9g

## Roasted Beet Pasta with Kale and Pesto

Time to prepare: 15 minutes
Time to cook: 10 minutes
Servings: 3

**Ingredients:**

For the Pesto:

- 1 large garlic clove, minced
- 3 cups fresh basil leaves
- 1/4 cup organic olive oil
- Salt & freshly ground black pepper to taste

For the Beet Pasta:

- 2 medium beets, trimmed, peeled, & spiralized
- Olive oil cooking spray
- Salt & freshly ground black pepper to taste

For the Kale:

- 2 cups fresh baby kale

**Directions:**

1. Preheat the oven to 425 degrees Fahrenheit and lightly grease a sizable baking sheet.
2. Blend the pesto ingredients in a blender until well combined. Set apart.
3. Set the prepared baking sheet with the beet pasta on it. Add salt and black pepper, then drizzle with cooking spray. Toss gently to evenly coat.
4. Roast for 5 to 10 minutes, depending on the desired level of doneness. Pasta should be moved to a big bowl. Add the pesto and kale. Serve after gently tossing to thoroughly coat.
**Nutritional Info:** Calories: 288; Fat: 28.8g; Carbs: 7.4g; Protein: 3.1g; Fiber: 2.9g

## Veggies and Aple with Orange Sauce

Time to prepare: 15 minutes
Time to cook: 16 minutes
Servings: 4
**Ingredients:**
For the Sauce:
- 2 garlic cloves, minced
- 1 (1 inch) fresh ginger, minced
- 1/2 cup fresh orange juice
- 1 tablespoon fresh orange zest, grated finely
- 2 tablespoon white wine vinegar
- 2 tablespoon coconut aminos
- 1 tablespoon red boat fish sauce

For the Veggies and Apple:
- 2 apples, cored & sliced
- 1 cup carrot, peeled & julienned
- 1 cup celery, chopped
- 1 cup onion, chopped
- 1 tablespoon extra-virgin olive oil

**Directions:**
1. Combine all the sauce ingredients in a large bowl. Set apart.
2. Heat the oil in your large skillet over medium-high heat. Stir-fry the carrot for approximately 4 minutes after adding it.
3. Stir-fry the celery and onion for about 4–5 minutes after adding them. Pour the sauce in, give it a good stir, and cook for two to three minutes.
4. Add the apple slices and cook for an additional 2–3 minutes. Serve warm.
**Nutritional Info:** Calories: 157; Fat: 4g; Carbs: 29.3g; Protein: 2g; Fiber: 3.6g

## Turkey Burgers

Time to prepare: 15 minutes
Time to cook: 16 minutes
Servings: 5
**Ingredients:**
- 1 lb. lean ground turkey
- 5 oz low-fat Halloumi cheese, grated
- 2 eggs
- 1 tablespoon fresh rosemary, chopped finely
- 1 tablespoon fresh parsley, chopped finely
- Salt & ground black pepper to taste

**Directions:**
1. Grease the grill grate and heat the grill to a medium-high temperature.
2. Combine all the ingredients in a big bowl and stir until everything is incorporated. From the ingredients, form 10 patties of the same size.
3. Add the hamburgers to the grill and cook for 5-8 minutes on each side, or until fully cooked.
**Nutritional Info:** Calories: 208; Fat: 10.3g; Carbs: 1g; Protein: 28g; Fiber: 0.2g

## Pasta with Cheesy Tomato Sauce

Time to prepare: 20 minutes
Time to cook: 55 minutes
Servings: 8
**Ingredients:**
- 1 large egg, lightly beaten
- 3 cups refined pasta, cooked & drained
- 1¾ cup tomato sauce, divided

- 1½ cup part-skim mozzarella cheese, shredded & divided
- 1 cup low-fat cottage cheese
- ½ teaspoon dried oregano
- Salt & ground black pepper to taste

**Directions:**

1. Grease an 8-inch square baking dish and preheat the oven to 375°F.

2. In the meantime, combine 3/4 cup tomato sauce, 1 cup mozzarella, cottage cheese, egg, dried herbs, and black pepper in a large dish. Add the spaghetti and mix well to coat.

3. Spread 1/4 cup of the prepared tomato sauce in the bottom of the baking dish.Add the pasta mixture, the remaining sauce, and the mozzarella cheese on top.

4. Bake for 45 minutes with the cover on. Bake for a further 5–10 minutes with the lid off. Serve warm.

**Nutritional Info:** Calories: 179; Fat: 2.6g; Carbs: 27.5g; Protein: 10.5g; Fiber: 2g

## Pasta With ucchini & Tomatoes

Time to prepare: 15 minutes
Time to cook: 20 minutes
Servings: 8

**Ingredients:**

- 3 tomatoes
- 1 lb. refined pasta
- 1 lb. zucchini, peeled, seeded & sliced
- ¾ cup low-fat feta cheese, crumbled
- ¼ cup olive oil
- 1 tablespoon garlic
- 1 teaspoon dried oregano, crushed
- Salt to taste
- Water, as needed

**Directions:**

1. Add the tomatoes to the boiling, salted water in your big pan and simmer for approximately a minute. With the slotted spoon, place the tomatoes in the dish of cold water.

2. Include the pasta in the boiling water in the same pan and cook for 8 to 10

minutes. the spaghetti thoroughly.

3. In the meantime, coarsely slice the peeled, seeded, and blanched tomatoes.

4. In a large pan, heat the oil over medium heat. Sauté the zucchini and garlic for approximately 4 minutes.

5. After the oregano and tomatoes have been added, simmer for 3–4 minutes. Mix the spaghetti and cheese together after adding them. Serve warm.

**Nutritional Info:** Calories: 272; Fat: 10.5g; Carbs: 25.3g; Protein: 9.5g; Fiber: 1.3g

## Chicken & Apple Lettuce Wraps

Time to prepare: 15 minutes
Time to cook: 0 minutes
Servings: 2-4

**Ingredients:**

- 1 seedless cucumber, sliced thinly
- 6 oz. cooked chicken breast, cut into strips
- ½ cup apple, peeled, cored & sliced thinly
- 4 large lettuce leaves
- 1 tablespoon fresh mint leaves, minced

**Directions:**

1. Combine all the ingredients, except the lettuce leaves, in a large bowl.

2. Arrange the lettuce leaves on plates for serving. Spread the chicken mixture equally over each lettuce leaf before serving.

**Nutritional Info:** Calories: 165; Fat: 2.9g; Carbs: 8.8g; Protein: 26g; Fiber: 1.7g

## Cheesy Chicken Meatballs

Time to prepare: 15 minutes
Time to cook: 10 minutes
Servings: 5

**Ingredients:**

- 1 large egg, beaten

- 1 lb. ground chicken
- ½ cup low-fat Parmesan cheese, grated freshly
- 4 tablespoon fresh parsley, chopped
- 2 tablespoon olive oil
- Salt & ground black pepper to taste

**Directions:**

1. In a large bowl, thoroughly combine all the ingredients, with the exception of the oil, using your hands. From the mixture, form little balls of equal size.

2. Heat the oil in a nonstick sauté pan over medium heat. Cook the meatballs for about 10 minutes, flipping them once or twice. Serve warm.

**Nutritional Info:** Calories: 262; Fat: 15.3g; Carbs: 0.4g; Protein: 26.9g; Fiber: 0.1g

## Beef & Mozzarella Burgers

Time to prepare: 15 minutes
Time to cook: 10 minutes
Servings: 2

**Ingredients:**

- 8 oz lean ground beef
- 1 oz part-skim mozzarella cheese, cubed
- 1 tablespoon olive oil
- Salt & ground black pepper to taste

**Directions:**

1. To a bowl, add the beef, salt, and black pepper, and stir to thoroughly combine. The mixture should be divided into two equal patties.

2. Before covering with beef, place a cube of mozzarella inside each patty.

3. Place your frying pan over medium heat, add the oil, and cook the patties for about 3 to 5 minutes on each side. Serve warm.

**Nutritional Info:** Calories: 311; Fat: 16.6g; Carbs: 0.5g; Protein: 38.4g; Fiber: 0g

## Tuna Stuffed Avocado

Time to prepare: 10 minutes
Time to cook: 0 minutes
Servings: 2

**Ingredients:**

- 1 large avocado, halved and pitted
- 1 (5-oz.) can of water-packed tuna, drained & flaked
- 3 tablespoon fat-free plain yogurt
- 2 tablespoon fresh lemon juice
- 1 teaspoon fresh parsley, chopped finely
- Salt & ground black pepper to taste

**Directions:**

1. Gently scoop out a couple tablespoons of flesh from each avocado half. Place the avocado halves on a platter and squeeze 1 teaspoon of lemon juice over each.

2. Cut the avocado flesh into small pieces and place it in a bowl. Stir in the tuna, yogurt, parsley, salt, black pepper, and any additional lemon juice.

3. Evenly distribute the tuna mixture between the two avocado halves. Serve right away.

**Nutritional Info:** Calories: 215; Fat: 11.8g; Carbs: 7g; Protein: 20.6g; Fiber: 3.2g

## Shrimp Lettuce Wraps

Time to prepare: 10 minutes
Time to cook: 4 minutes
Servings: 6

**Ingredients:**

- 1½ lb. shrimp, peeled, deveined & chopped
- 12 butter lettuce leaves
- 1 cup carrot, peeled & julienned
- 1 tablespoon extra-virgin olive oil
- Salt & ground black pepper to taste

**Directions:**

1. In a large pan, heat the oil over medium heat. Add the shrimp and cook for 3 to 4 minutes, seasoning with salt and black

pepper. Place aside.

2. Distribute the lettuce leaves among the dishes. Sprinkle the shrimp and carrot equally over the lettuce leaves. Serve right away.

**Nutritional Info:** Calories: 164; Fat: 4.3g; Carbs: 3.8g; Protein: 26g; Fiber:0.5g

### Fried Rice with Kale

Time to prepare: 10 minutes
Time to cook: 12 minutes
Servings: 2

**Ingredients:**
- 3 sliced scallions
- 1 ½ cup cooked white rice
- 1 cup kale, stemmed & chopped
- 2 tablespoon stir-fry sauce
- 1 tablespoon extra-virgin olive oil

**Directions:**
1. In a large skillet over medium-high heat, warm the olive oil. Add the greens and scallions. Cook the veggies until they are soft.
2. In a mixing bowl, combine the brown rice and stir-fry sauce. Cook while frequently stirring until well heated. Serve!

**Nutritional Info:** Calories: 308; Fat: 11.3g; Carbs: 41.9g; Protein: 9.5g; Fiber: 4.38 g

### Shrimp & Tomato Bake

Time to prepare: 15 minutes
Time to cook: 27 minutes
Servings: 6

**Ingredients:**
- 1½ lb. large shrimp, peeled and deveined
- ½ cup homemade chicken broth
- 2 cups tomatoes, peeled, seeded & chopped
- ¼ cup fresh parsley, chopped
- 4 oz low-fat feta cheese, crumbled
- 2 tablespoon olive oil

- ¾ teaspoon dried oregano, crushed

**Directions:**
1. Set the oven to 350°F.
2. In your sauté pan, heat the oil to medium-high heat before adding the oregano and cooking the shrimp for about 2 minutes.
3. Add the parsley and salt, then quickly and evenly pour into a casserole dish.
4. Place the broth in the same pan and heat it over medium-low for about 2–3 minutes, or until it has reduced by half. Cook for two to three minutes after adding the tomatoes.
5. Evenly distribute the tomato mixture over the shrimp mixture, then sprinkle cheese on top.
6. Bake for 15 to 20 minutes, or until the top is browned. Serve warm.

**Nutritional Info:** Calories: 150; Fat: 7g; Carbs: 5.4g; Protein: 25.7g; Fiber: 0.9g

### Lemony Scallops

Time to prepare: 10 minutes
Time to cook: 5 minutes
Servings: 4

**Ingredients:**
- 1 lb. sea scallops
- 2 tablespoon olive oil
- 2 tablespoon fresh rosemary, chopped
- 1 tablespoon fresh lemon juice
- ½ teaspoon lemon zest, grated
- Salt & ground black pepper to taste

**Directions:**
1. In a medium sauté pan, heat the oil over medium-high heat before adding the lemon zest and rosemary.
2. Include the scallops and cook them for two minutes on each side. Serve hot after adding salt, black pepper, and lemon juice.

**Nutritional Info:** Calories: 166; Fat: 8.1g; Carbs: 3.9g; Protein: 19.2g; Fiber: 0.7g

# DINNER

## Stuffed Zucchini Boats

Time to prepare: 15 minutes
Time to cook: 30 minutes
Servings: 3-6

**Ingredients:**

- 1 lb. ground turkey
- 1 (28 oz) can crush tomatoes
- 6 large zucchinis, divide half lengthwise & scoop out the seeds
- 2 garlic cloves, minced
- 1 small yellow onion, diced
- 4 oz Mozzarella cheese, shredded
- 1 oz Parmesan cheese, freshly grated
- 1/2 tablespoon olive oil
- 1/4 teaspoon garlic powder
- Flat-leaf parsley for garnishing
- Kosher salt & ground black pepper to taste
- Cooking spray

**Directions:**

1. Preheat your oven to 425°F and spray cooking spray in a 9- by 13-inch baking dish to lightly grease it.
2. After seasoning the zucchini with salt, pepper, and garlic powder, brush it with olive oil. It should start to soften after 20 minutes of roasting in the prepared dish.
3. Meanwhile, sauté the onions and garlic in 1/2 tablespoon olive oil in a large skillet over medium-high heat.
4. After cooking for 3 to 4 minutes, add the ground turkey and cook it. Let the tomatoes boil after adding them.
5. Make the heat medium and cook the zucchini for the desired amount of time. Add a half-teaspoon of salt and pepper, to taste.
6. Bake for no more than five minutes, or until the mozzarella cheese is melted. Serve hot with parsley and Parmesan cheese as garnishes.

**Nutritional Info:** Calories: 173; Fat: 17.1g; Carbs: 10.5g; Protein: 14.2g; Fiber: 3.6g

## Roasted Salmon and Asparagus

Time to prepare: 10 minutes
Time to cook: 15 minutes
Servings: 2

**Ingredients:**

- 1 lb. salmon, cut into two fillets
- 1/2 lb. asparagus spears, trimmed
- 1/2 lemon zest and slices
- 1 tablespoon extra-virgin olive oil
- 1 teaspoon sea salt, divided
- 1/8 teaspoon freshly cracked black pepper

**Directions:**

1. Preheat the oven to 425°F.
2. Use half the salt and half the oil to season the asparagus. Add salt and pepper to the fish to season it. On your roasting pan, spread it out.
3. Place the asparagus on top and garnish with lemon slices and zest.
4. Roast the fish for about 15 minutes, or until it is opaque. Serve!

**Nutritional Info:** Calories: 507; Fat: 33.8g; Carbs: 4.4g; Protein: 48g; Fiber: 2.1g

## Chicken Cutlets

Time to prepare: 10 minutes
Time to cook: 5 minutes
Servings: 4

**Ingredients:**

- 1 lb. chicken breast cutlets
- 1/4 cup refined white flour
- 4 teaspoon red wine vinegar
- 2 teaspoon minced garlic cloves
- 2 teaspoon dried sage leaves

- 2 teaspoon olive oil
- Salt & pepper to taste

**Directions:**

1. Spread a piece of plastic wrap on the kitchen surface and sprinkle with half the mixture of vinegar, sage, and garlic.

2. Spread the plastic wrap over the chicken breast and sprinkle with the remaining vinegar mixture. Add salt and pepper sparingly.

3. Cover the chicken with the second plastic wrap sheet to keep it safe. The breast should be flattened with a kitchen mallet. Observe it for five minutes.

4. Sprinkle flour over the chicken's top and bottom.

5. Heat the oil in a skillet over medium heat. Add the first half of the chicken breast and heat for 1 1/2 minutes, or until the bottom is browned.

6. Flip it over and cook for another three minutes. Repeat with the remaining cutlets after removing and setting them aside.

**Nutritional Info:** Calories: 189; Fat: 5.5g; Carbs: 6.63g; Protein: 26.4g; Fiber: 0.2g

### Halibut Curry

Time to prepare: 10 minutes
Time to cook: 9 minutes
Servings: 2

**Ingredients:**

- 1 lb. halibut, skin & bones removed, cut into 1-inch pieces
- 1/2 (14 oz) canned coconut milk
- 2 cups of no-salt-added chicken broth
- 1 tablespoon extra-virgin olive oil
- 1 teaspoon ground turmeric
- 1/8 teaspoon ground black pepper
- 1 teaspoon curry powder
- 1/4 teaspoon sea salt

**Directions:**

1. In a nonstick skillet over medium-high heat, warm the olive oil.

2. In a bowl, combine the curry powder and the turmeric. Cook the spices in your pan while turning often for 2 minutes to bloom the flavors.

3. Add the salt, pepper, coconut milk, and chicken broth. Set the heat to medium-low and let it simmer. Cook the salmon for 6–7 minutes, or until it becomes opaque. Serve!

**Nutritional Info:** Calories: 373; Fat: 31g; Carbs: 5g; Protein: 21.6g; Fiber: 1g

### Vegetable Pate with White Rice Cakes

Time to prepare: 20 minutes
Time to cook: 10 minutes
Servings: 4

**Ingredients:**

For the Korean rice cakes:

- 1 egg beaten
- 1 cup cooked white sticky rice
- ½ teaspoon Himalayan salt
- 1 teaspoon coconut oil

For the veggie pate:

- 1 cup cooked zucchini, peeled & deseeded
- 1 cup cooked beet, peeled & deseeded
- 1 cup cooked pumpkin, peeled & deseeded
- 4 tablespoon cottage or other soft cheese, grated
- 2 teaspoon coconut oil, divided
- 2 teaspoon smooth peanut butter
- 1 teaspoon garlic powder, divided
- 2 teaspoon dried Italian herbs (thyme, rosemary), divided
- 1 teaspoon fresh cilantro finely chopped
- 1 teaspoon fresh basil or mint finely chopped
- Himalayan salt, to taste

**Directions:**

1. In your bowl, combine the rice, egg, and Himalayan salt. Form 4 sizing-

appropriate balls from this mixture by kneading it, then flatten each into a patty.

2. In a frying pan with hot oil, cook the rice cakes for 4 to 5 minutes on each side, or until crisp and golden brown.

3. In a basin, mash the beet, pumpkin, and zucchini. Put the cheese and vegetables in four different dishes.

4. Distribute the herbs, smooth peanut butter, Himalayan salt, and garlic powder evenly among the four bowls, then thoroughly combine. Give one pate mix to each rice cake.

**Nutritional Info:** Calories: 173; Fat: 5.5g; Carbs: 27.5g; Protein: 4g; Fiber: 2.2g

## Rosemary Chicken

Time to prepare: 15 minutes
Time to cook: 20 minutes
Servings: 2

**Ingredients:**
- 1 lb. chicken breast tenders
- 1 tablespoon chopped fresh rosemary leaves
- 1 tablespoon extra-virgin olive oil
- 1/8 teaspoon ground black pepper
- 1/4 teaspoon sea salt

**Directions:**
1. Preheat the oven to 425°F.
2. Arrange the chicken tenders on a rimmed baking sheet. Salt, rosemary, and pepper oil are sprinkled on top after they have been brushed with oil.
3. Bake the food for 15 to 20 minutes, or until the juices flow clearly. Serve!

**Nutritional Info:** Calories: 336; Fat: 13.1g; Carbs: 0.3g; Protein: 51g; Fiber: 0.1g

## Lemony Salmon

Time to prepare: 10 minutes
Time to cook: 14 minutes
Servings: 4

**Ingredients:**
- 4 (6-oz.) boneless, skinless salmon fillets
- 1 tablespoon fresh lemon zest, grated
- 2 tablespoon extra-virgin olive oil
- 2 tablespoon fresh lemon juice
- Salt & freshly ground black pepper to taste

**Directions:**
1. Grease the grill grate and heat the grill to a medium-high temperature.
2. Combine all the ingredients, excluding the salmon fillets, in a medium bowl. Add the salmon fillets and generously brush them with the garlic mixture.
3. Put the salmon fillets on the grill and cook them for about 6–7 minutes per side. Serve warm.

**Nutritional Info:** Calories: 383; Fat: 27g; Carbs: 0.9g; Protein: 34.5g; Fiber: 0.2g

## Asian Tofu Stir Fry

Time to prepare: 10 minutes
Time to cook: 7 minutes
Servings: 2-3

**Ingredients:**
- 1 (8 oz) packet rice noodles, cooked
- 1 roasted red bell pepper, deseeded & thinly sliced (if tolerated)
- 1 cup tofu, cubed
- 1 cup canned green beans, halved
- 2 tablespoon soy sauce
- 2 tablespoon coconut oil
- ¼ cup spring onions greens

**Directions:**
1. In your saucepan, heat the oil to a medium-high temperature. Sauté the green parts of the spring onions for one to two minutes on medium heat.
2. Add the vegetables and tofu, and stir-fry for 4-5 minutes on high heat. Soy sauce and noodles together After removing from the heat, serve.

**Nutritional Info:** Calories: 221; Fat: 6.4g; Carbs: 29.3g; Protein: 11.3g; Fiber: 2.3g

## Gingered Turkey Meatballs

Time to prepare: 15 minutes
Time to cook: 10 minutes
Servings: 2

**Ingredients:**
- 1 lb. ground turkey
- 2 tablespoon chopped fresh cilantro leaves
- 1/2 tablespoon grated fresh ginger
- 1/2 teaspoon onion powder
- 1/2 teaspoon garlic powder
- 1/4 teaspoon sea salt
- 1 tablespoon olive oil
- A pinch of freshly ground black pepper

**Directions:**
1. Combine the turkey, cilantro, ginger, onion, garlic, pepper, and salt in a large bowl. The turkey mixture should be formed into 10 meatballs.
2. In a sizable nonstick skillet, heat the oil over medium-high heat. The meatballs should be cooked for about 10 minutes, rotating them as they brown. Serve!

**Nutritional Info:** Calories: 559; Fat: 47.6g; Carbs: 4.5g; Protein: 28.8g; Fiber: 0.7g

## Herbed Salmon

Time to prepare: 10 minutes + marinating time
Time to cook: 8 minutes
Servings: 4

**Ingredients:**
- 4 (4-oz.) salmon fillets
- ¼ cup olive oil
- 2 tablespoon fresh lemon juice
- 1 teaspoon dried oregano, crushed
- 1 teaspoon dried basil, crushed

- Salt & freshly ground black pepper to taste

**Directions:**
1. Combine all the ingredients in a large bowl, excluding the salmon. Add the salmon and generously cover it with the marinade.
2. Cover and place in the refrigerator for at least an hour to marinate. Grease the grill grate and heat the grill to a medium-high temperature.
3. Place the salmon on your grill, cooking it for about 4 minutes on each side. Serve warm.

**Nutritional Info:** Calories: 341; Fat: 27.6g; Carbohydrates: 1.0g; Protein: 23g; Fiber: 0.3g

## Cantaloupe Gnocchi

Time to prepare: 10 minutes
Time to cook: 4-6 minutes
Servings: 4

**Ingredients:**
- 4-5 cups cantaloupe, skinned. cut into chunks, & steamed
- 2 cups refined flour
- 1 teaspoon olive oil
- Himalayan salt to taste
- Water, as needed

**Directions:**
1. Combine the flour and steamed cantaloupe in a big bowl. For a doughy mixture, thoroughly stir and knead the ingredients. Hand-roll several gnocchi-shaped pieces, then save them.
2. Bring a pot of water to a boil, add your gnocchi pieces, and cook for 4-6 minutes, or until they float to the surface. Cleanly drain, then plate!

**Nutritional Info:** Calories: 305; Fat: 2.2g; Carbs: 58.1g; Protein: 9.1g; Fiber: 2.2g

## Veggie Risotto

Time to prepare: 10 minutes
Time to cook: 23 minutes
Servings: 2

**Ingredients:**

- 1 cup white risotto rice, cooked
- 1 cup grated zucchini, peeled & deseeded
- 1 cup water
- ½ cup canned green beans halved
- 1 tablespoon extra virgin olive oil
- 1 teaspoon apple cider vinegar
- 1 teaspoon dried basil
- A sprig of parsley, finely chopped
- Himalayan salt to taste
- Herbs for garnish

**Directions:**

1. Within 6 to 8 minutes, fry the vegetables in the oil in your skillet until they begin to soften and brown.
2. Include the rice, water, herbs, and apple cider vinegar. It needs to be cooked for 15 minutes to taste right. Serve with fresh herbs as a garnish.

**Nutritional Info:** Calories: 142; Fat: 3.4g; Carbs: 25.5g; Protein: 2.9g; Fiber: 1.3g

## Lemon Pepper Turkey

Time to prepare: 10 minutes
Time to cook: 20 minutes
Servings: 4

**Ingredients:**

- 1 lb. turkey breasts, boneless & skinless halved
- 2 lemons, divided (1 zested & 1 sliced)
- 2 minced cloves of garlic
- ½ cup refined flour
- ½ cup chicken broth
- 4 tablespoon olive oil
- 1 tablespoon lemon pepper seasoning
- 1 teaspoon kosher salt

**Directions:**

1. Preheat the oven to 400F.
2. Combine flour, salt, lemon pepper, and the zest of one lemon in a bowl. Add the turkey and thoroughly coat.
3. Cook the turkey for 5 minutes on one side in heated oil.
4. Combine the remaining ingredients and bake for the last 15 minutes. Serve.

**Nutritional Info:** Calories 231; Fat 6g; Carbs 12g; Protein 14g; Fiber 1.7g

## Baked Pumpkin Risotto

Time to prepare: 15 minutes
Time to cook: 40 minutes
Servings: 2

**Ingredients:**

- 1 carrot, peeled & shredded
- 1 cup arborio or white risotto rice
- 2½ cups vegetable stock
- 2 cups grated pumpkin
- 1 cup shredded green lettuce
- 1 sprig basil
- ½ garlic clove (if tolerated)
- 4 tablespoon cottage cheese
- 2 teaspoon extra virgin olive oil
- Pinch of pink Himalayan salt

**Directions:**

1. Turn on the oven to 400°F.
2. Set your pan's oil to medium heat. After the garlic has been browned for two minutes, add the pumpkin, carrot, basil, and Himalayan salt, and cook for six to eight minutes more.
3. Move it to a baking dish, then incorporate the rice and stock. 30 minutes into baking, remove from oven, and stir in cottage cheese. Serve!

**Nutritional Info:** Calories: 240; Carbs: 38.4g; Fat: 7.8g; Protein: 4.8g; Fiber: 4g

## Pasta Puttanesca

Time to prepare: 15 minutes
Time to cook: 20 minutes
Servings: 4

**Ingredients:**
- 1 (8 oz) white pasta of choice, cooked & drained
- 1 roasted red bell pepper, deseeded & julienned (if tolerated)
- 1 beet, peeled & julienned, squeezed
- 1 tablespoon olive oil
- 2 cups tomato puree
- 2 tablespoon canned capers or artichoke hearts
- 1 tablespoon tomato paste (optional)
- 2 teaspoon Italian seasoning
- 1 teaspoon salt

**Directions:**
1. In a saucepan over medium heat, heat the oil, then sauté the vegetables for 6 to 8 minutes, or until they are soft.
2. Cook the tomato puree for 8 to 10 minutes on medium-low heat with the capers, salt, seasoning, and tomato paste (if using).
3. Include the pasta and combine by stirring. Prepare in one to two minutes over low heat and serve.

**Nutritional Info:** Calories: 301; Carbs: 48g; Fat: 4.5g; Protein: 7.2g; Fiber: 2.1g

## Chicken Piccata

Time to prepare: 10 minutes
Time to cook: 20 minutes
Servings: 4

**Ingredients:**
- 3 chicken breasts, sliced into 6 cutlets
- 2 garlic cloves, minced
- 2 lemons' juice
- 1 lemon, sliced
- 2 cups chicken stock
- 1 cup all-purpose flour
- 1/4 cup capers
- 1/3 cup white wine
- 6 tablespoon olive oil
- Granulated garlic, to taste
- Salt & pepper to taste

**Directions:**
Granulated garlic, salt, and pepper are used to season the cutlets. Spread the flour over them.
1. Heat the olive oil in your pan, then add the chicken cutlets and cook for 4 minutes on each side. Dispatch it on a plate.
2. Brown the garlic in the same pan while also adding the lemon slices, garlic granules, salt, pepper, stock, and wine.
3. After letting it come to a boil, add the chicken and capers and cook for 5 minutes. Serve.

**Nutritional Info:** Calories 276; Fat 15g; Carbs 14g; Protein 17g; Fiber 1g

## Whole Roasted Trout

Time to prepare: 10 minutes
Time to cook: 16 minutes
Servings: 2

**Ingredients:**
- 1/2 lb. whole trout
- 1 lemon, sliced
- 6 sprigs of fresh thyme
- ½ shallot, thinly sliced
- 1 tablespoon olive oil
- 4 teaspoon butter, cubed (if tolerated)
- Salt & black pepper to taste

**Directions:**
1. Oven temperature: 425 °F.
2. Oil the fish and sprinkle it with salt and pepper.
3. Place the chicken, skin side down, on a baking sheet coated with aluminum, and then cover with the other ingredients.
4. After baking for 12 to 16 minutes, serve.

**Nutritional Info:** Calories 178; Fat 6g; Carbs 13g; Protein 14.3g; Fiber 2g

## Sriracha Lime Chicken Apple & Tomato Salad

Time to prepare: 10 minutes

Time to cook: 28 minutes
Servings: 4
**Ingredients:**
For the Sriracha Lime Chicken:
- 2 organic chicken breasts
- 3 tablespoon sriracha
- 1 lime, juiced
- 1/4 teaspoon fine sea salt
- 1/4 teaspoon freshly ground pepper
- 4 apples, peeled, cored, & diced

For the Salad:
- 1 cup organic grape tomatoes, peeled & seeded
- 1/3 cup red onion, finely chopped (if tolerated)

For the Lime Vinaigrette:
- 1/3 cup light olive oil
- 1/4 cup apple cider vinegar
- 2 limes, juiced
- A dash of fine sea salt

**Directions:**
1. Add salt and pepper to the chicken's seasoning. Apply the Sriracha and lime, then let it stand for 20 minutes.
2. In a skillet with oil over medium heat, cook the chicken for 3 minutes on each side, or until done. Cook the apple for two minutes after adding it.
3. In the meantime, combine the ingredients for the lime vinaigrette in a basin. Place aside.
4. Combine the tomatoes and red onion in a bowl, and then pour the dressing over the top. Dispense with the chicken and apple as a side dish.
**Nutritional Info:** Calories: 467; Fat: 29.1g; Carbs: 27.8gl Protein: 25g; Fiber: 3.2g


## Scallops with Lemon-Ginger Vinaigrette

Time to prepare: 10 minutes
Time to cook: 6 minutes

Servings: 2
**Ingredients:**
- 1 lb. sea scallops
- 2 tablespoon lemon-ginger vinaigrette
- 1 tablespoon extra-virgin olive oil
- 1/4 teaspoon sea salt
- A pinch of freshly ground black pepper

**Directions:**
1. In a nonstick skillet or pan, heat the olive oil over medium-high heat.
2. Add the scallops to the skillet, season with salt and pepper, and cook for 3 minutes on each side, or until the fish is just opaque. Add a dollop of vinaigrette before serving.
**Nutritional Info:** Calories: 312; Fat: 18g; Carbs: 7.8g; Protein: 29g; Fiber: 0g


## Portobello Mushroom Pizza

Time to prepare: 10 minutes
Time to cook: 20 minutes
Servings: 1
**Ingredients:**
- 1 portobello mushroom
- ½ cup marinara sauce (if tolerated), or homemade tomato sauce
- 1 oz mozzarella cheese

**Directions:**
1. Oven temperature: 425 °F.
2. Scrape out the interior of the mushroom, then combine the sauce with the mushroom flesh. Place cheese on top of this mixture after pouring it inside the mushroom.
3. Bake for 20 minutes, then let it cool before serving.
**Nutritional Info:** Calories 133; Fat 6g; Protein 10g; Carbs 11g; Fiber 1.2g


## Turkey and Kale Sauté

Time to prepare: 15 minutes

Time to cook: 35 minutes
Servings: 2
**Ingredients:**
- 1 lb. ground turkey breast
- 3 minced garlic cloves
- 1/2 chopped onion
- 1 cup stemmed and chopped kale
- 1/2 teaspoon sea salt
- 1 tablespoon extra-virgin olive oil
- 1 tablespoon fresh thyme leaves
- A pinch of freshly ground black pepper

**Directions:**
1. In a large nonstick skillet over medium-high heat, warm the olive oil until it shimmers.
2. Include the kale, onion, thyme, pepper, and salt with the turkey. Cook the turkey for 5 minutes, breaking it up with a spoon as it browns.
3. After adding the garlic, simmer it for 30 minutes while stirring constantly. Serve!

**Nutritional Info:** Calories: 342; Fat: 9.58g; Carbs: 7g; Protein: 58.7g; Fiber: 1.6g

## Southeastern Seasoned Catfish

Time to prepare: 10 minutes
Time to cook: 9 minutes
Servings: 2
**Ingredients:**
- 2 catfish fillets, boneless & skinless
- 2 teaspoon dried minced onion
- ½ teaspoon paprika (if tolerated)
- ½ teaspoon garlic powder
- 1/4 teaspoon mustard powder
- 1/4 teaspoon cayenne pepper
- Cooking spray

**Directions:**
1. Place all the ingredients in a dish, except the fish and frying spray. Apply this mixture to the fish, coating it well.
2. Place the fish on top of the oil-spraying-coated baking sheet. Broil for 5 minutes, then flip and broil for an additional 3 to 4 minutes. Serve!

**Nutritional Info:** Calories 239; Fat 14g; Carbs 0g; Protein 27g; Fiber 1 g

## Winter Apple Poke Bowl

Time to prepare: 10 minutes
Time to cook: 50 minutes
Servings: 2
**Ingredients:**
- 1 packet of precooked white rice
- 1 red apple, peeled & sliced
- ½ butternut pumpkin, peeled, seeded & chopped
- 7 oz diced halloumi
- ½ cup parsley & coriander
- ½ cup chopped chives
- 2 tablespoon lemon juice
- 2 tablespoon olive oil
- 1 tablespoon organic honey
- 1 teaspoon grated ginger

**Directions:**
1. Preheat the oven to 390°F. To make the pumpkin tender, roast it for 30 to 40 minutes. Halloumi should be cooked in a pan until golden.
2. Place the remaining ingredients in a bowl, then top with the roasted pumpkin and halloumi. Serve

**Nutritional Info:** Calories 178; Fat 4g; Carbs 14g; Protein 3g; Fiber 4g

## Creamy Tuscan Chicken Pasta

Time to prepare: 10 minutes
Time to cook: 14 minutes
Servings: 4
**Ingredients:**
- 1 1/2 lb. diced chicken breast, boneless & skinless

- 10 oz short refined pasta, cooked & drained
- 8 oz sun-dried (in oil) tomatoes, chopped
- 3-4 garlic cloves, minced
- 3 cups almond milk
- 3 cups baby spinach
- ½ cup Parmesan cheese
- 2 tablespoon flour
- 2 tablespoon olive oil
- 1 teaspoon Italian seasoning
- Salt & pepper to taste

**Directions:**

1. In a bowl, combine the chicken with the Italian seasoning, oil, garlic, salt, and pepper. For two to three minutes, cook the chicken in a skillet with a drizzle of heated oil.

2. After adding the tomatoes, simmer for 5 to 7 minutes.

3. Whisk together the milk and flour in a mixing bowl. Heat for three to four minutes in your pan. Pasta with cheese should be added before serving.

**Nutritional Info:** Calories 368; Fat 13g; Carbs 36g; Protein 27g; Fiber 4g

## French Oven Beef Stew

Time to prepare: 10 minutes
Time to cook: 4 hours
Servings: 6

**Ingredients:**
- 1 lb. stew beef, sliced into cubes
- 6 carrots, peeled & chopped
- 4 parsnips, peeled & chopped
- 4 potatoes, peeled & chopped
- 1 cup of diced fennel bulb
- 1 celery stalk
- 1 cup tomato juice, no seeds
- 1/4 cup quick-cooking tapioca
- 1 tablespoon stevia
- 1 teaspoon ground basil
- ½ teaspoon each of salt & black pepper

**Directions:**

1. Preheat the oven to 300F.

2. Except for the potatoes, add all the fixings to your large shallow baking dish and bake for three hours.

3. Include the potatoes, and bake for an additional hour. Serve.

**Nutritional Info:** Calories 213; Fat 8g; Carbs 16g; Protein 30g; Fiber 2g

## Prawn & Tomato Spaghetti

Time to prepare: 20 minutes
Time to cook: 6 minutes
Servings: 6

**Ingredients:**
- 20 green prawns, peeled & deveined
- 6 tomatoes, peeled, seeded & chopped
- 4 garlic cloves, sliced
- 13 oz refined spaghetti, cooked & drained
- 2 tablespoon chopped parsley leaves
- 1 tablespoon olive oil

**Directions:**

1. In a pan with hot oil, sauté the garlic for one minute over medium heat.

2. Include the prawns and cook for two to three minutes. Cook for 2 minutes after adding the tomatoes.

3. Combine the pasta and parsley by tossing. Serve!

**Nutritional Info:** Calories 490; Fat 6.5g; Carbs 50g; Protein 33g; Fiber 1.2g

## Orange and Maple-Glazed Salmon

Time to prepare: 10 minutes
Time to cook: 15 minutes
Servings: 2

**Ingredients:**
- 2 (4-6 oz) salmon fillets, pin bones removed
- 1 orange, zested & juiced
- 2 tablespoon pure maple syrup
- 1 tablespoon low-sodium soy sauce

- 1 teaspoon garlic powder

**Directions:**

1. Preheat the oven to 400°F.
2. In a small bowl, combine the orange juice, zest, soy sauce, maple syrup, and garlic powder.
3. Place the salmon flesh-side down on the serving plate. Give it 10 minutes to marinate.
4. Place the salmon skin-side up on a baking sheet and bake for 15 minutes, or until the flesh is opaque. Serve!

**Nutritional Info:** Calories: 297; Fat: 13.4g; Carbs: 20.8g; Protein: 24g; Fiber: 0.7g

### Chicken Cacciatore

Time to prepare: 10 minutes
Time to cook: 20 minutes
Servings: 2

**Ingredients:**

- 1 lb. skinless chicken, cut into bite-size pieces
- 1 (28 oz) can of crushed tomatoes, drained
- 1/4 cup black olives, chopped
- 1 tablespoon extra-virgin olive oil
- 1/2 teaspoon onion powder
- 1/2 teaspoon garlic powder
- 1/4 teaspoon sea salt
- A pinch of freshly ground black pepper

**Directions:**

1. In a nonstick skillet over medium-high heat, warm the olive oil. Cook the chicken until it turns golden.
2. Stir in the tomatoes, garlic powder, olive oil, salt, onion powder, and pepper. 10 minutes of stirring while cooking. Serve!

**Nutritional Info:** Calories: 343; Fat: 14.2g; Carbs: 20.2g; Protein: 39g; Fiber: 5.1g

### Peach Stew

Time to prepare: 10 minutes
Time to cook: 10 minutes
Servings: 6

**Ingredients:**

- 5 cups peeled and cubed peaches
- 2 cups water
- 3 tablespoon stevia
- 1 teaspoon grated ginger

**Directions:**

1. In a saucepan, mix the peaches, stevia, ginger, and water.
2. Combine thoroughly, simmer over medium heat for 10 minutes, then divide among bowls and serve cold.

**Nutritional Info:** Calories 142; Fat 1.5g; Carbs 7.8g; Protein 2.4g, Fiber 1.7g

### Shrimp Salmon Tomato Stew

Time to prepare: 10 minutes
Time to cook: 18 minutes
Servings: 8

**Ingredients:**

- 1 lb. salmon fillets, cubed
- 1 lb. shrimp, peeled and deveined
- 4 cups fish bone broth
- 2½ cup fresh tomatoes, peeled, seeded, & chopped
- 2 tablespoon fresh lime juice
- 3 tablespoon fresh parsley, chopped
- Salt & freshly ground black pepper to taste

**Directions:**

1. Stir the tomatoes and broth together in a big soup pot and bring to a boil. Set the heat to medium, then simmer for about five minutes.
2. Include the salmon and cook for 3 to 4 minutes. Add the shrimp, stir, and cook for about four to five minutes.
3. Remove from the heat and stir in the lemon juice, salt, and black pepper. Serve hot with parsley as a garnish.

**Nutritional Info:** Calories: 173; Fat: 5.5g; Carbs: 3.2g; Protein: 27.1g; Fiber: 0.7g

## Zero-Fiber Chicken Dish

Time to prepare: 5 minutes + marinating time
Time to cook: 10 minutes
Servings: 6
**Ingredients:**

- 4 (6-oz.) chicken breast halves, boneless, skinless
- 2 tablespoon olive oil
- Salt & freshly ground black pepper to taste

**Directions:**
1. Add salt and black pepper to each chicken.
2. Set the chicken breast halves over a rack that is positioned on a baking sheet with a rim. For at least 30 minutes, refrigerate. Remove and use paper towels to dry.
3. Heat the oil in your skillet over a medium-low flame. The chicken breast halves should be placed smooth-side down and cooked motionless for 9 to 10 minutes.
4. Cook the chicken breasts on the other side for about 6 minutes, or until done. Slice it after cooling, then serve!
**Nutritional Info:** Calories: 178; Fat: 7.7g; Carbs: 0.1g; Protein: 26g; Fiber: 0g

## Mushroom Goulash with Rice

Time to prepare: 10 minutes
Time to cook: 12 minutes
Servings: 2
**Ingredients:**

- 1 cup mushrooms of choice, halved
- 1 cup cooked white rice
- 1 small yellow pepper, deseeded & finely chopped (if tolerated)

- 1½ cup buttermilk
- ½ cup lettuce, shredded
- 1 tablespoon parsley leaves, chopped
- 2-3 teaspoon olive oil
- 1 teaspoon mustard
- 1 teaspoon salt

**Directions:**
1. Add the mushrooms to the hot olive oil in your large skillet.
2. Include the mustard, salt, and vegetables. Cook the mushrooms for 8 minutes or until they are fully cooked.
3. After adding the buttermilk, simmer the sauce for 3–4 minutes on low heat, or until it slightly thickens. Add some chopped parsley. Serve the goulash over overcooked rice.
**Nutritional Info:** Calories: 276; Fat: 7.1g; Carbs: 40.4g; Protein: 11.1g; Fiber: 1.6g

## Mushroom Chicken Platter

Time to prepare: 15 minutes
Time to cook: 17 minutes
Servings: 6
**Ingredients:**

- 4 (4-oz.) chicken breasts, boneless, skinless, cut into small pieces
- 4 cups fresh mushrooms, sliced
- 1 cups chicken bone broth
- 2 tablespoon olive oil, divided
- 1 teaspoon fresh ginger, grated
- Salt & freshly ground black pepper to taste

**Directions:**
1. Stir-fry the chicken pieces with salt, black pepper, and 1 tablespoon oil in a large pan over medium-high heat for approximately 4–5 minutes, or until golden brown.
2. Transfer the chicken pieces onto a dish using a slotted spoon.
3. In the same skillet, heat the remaining oil over medium heat and cook the onion and ginger for approximately a minute.

4. Add the mushrooms and simmer, stirring often, for approximately 6-7 minutes. Stir-fry for 3–4 minutes after adding the prepared chicken and coconut milk.

5. Add the salt and black pepper, then turn off the heat. Serve warm.

**Nutritional Info:** Calories: 200; Fat: 10.4g; Carbs: 1.6g; Protein: 24.8g; Fiber: 0.5g

## Easiest Tuna Salad

Time to prepare: 15 minutes
Time to cook: 0 minutes
Servings: 4
**Ingredients:**
For the Dressing:
- 2 tablespoon fresh dill, minced
- 2 tablespoon olive oil
- 1 tablespoon fresh lime juice
- Salt & freshly ground black pepper to taste

For the Salad:
- 2 (6-oz.) cans of water-packed tuna, drained and flaked
- 6 hard-boiled eggs, peeled and sliced
- 1 cup tomato, peeled, seeded, and chopped
- 1 large cucumber, peeled, seeded, and sliced

**Directions:**
1. In a bowl, combine all the dressing ingredients and whisk to combine.
2. Combine all the ingredients in a second big serving bowl.
3. Distribute the tuna mixture among plates for serving. Serve after the dressing is drizzled.

**Nutritional Info:** Calories: 277; Fat: 14.5g; Carbs: 5.9g; Protein: 31.2g; Fiber: 0.96g

## Prawns with Asparagus

Time to prepare: 15 minutes
Time to cook: 13 minutes
Servings: 5
**Ingredients:**
- 1 lb. prawns, peeled & deveined
- 1 lb. asparagus, trimmed
- 2 tablespoon olive oil
- 2 tablespoon fresh lemon juice
- 1 teaspoon fresh ginger, minced
- Salt & freshly ground black pepper to taste

**Directions:**
1. In a skillet, heat 1 tablespoon of oil over medium-high heat. Add the prawns and cook for about 3 to 4 minutes, seasoning with salt and black pepper.
2. Put the prawns in a bowl using a slotted spoon. Place aside.
3. In the same skillet, heat the remaining oil over medium-high heat. Add the asparagus, ginger, salt, and black pepper, and cook, stirring frequently, for about 6 to 8 minutes.
4. Add the prawns and stir; cook for about one minute. Serve hot after adding the lemon juice.

**Nutritional Info:** Calories: 127; Fat: 6.5g; Carbs: 3.5g; Protein: 14.3g; Fiber: 2.0g

## Chicken Salad Sandwiches

Time to prepare: 10 minutes
Time to cook: 0 minutes
Servings: 2
**Ingredients:**
- 4 slices of white bread
- 1 cup chicken, chopped, cooked, and skinless (from 1 rotisserie chicken)
- 2 tablespoon anti-inflammatory mayonnaise
- 1 tablespoon chopped fresh tarragon leaves

- 1/2 minced red bell pepper (if tolerated)
- 1 teaspoon Dijon mustard (if tolerated)
- 1/4 teaspoon sea salt

**Directions:**

1. In a medium bowl, mix the chicken, red bell pepper, mayonnaise, mustard, tarragon, and salt.

2. Spread on two pieces of bread, then cover them with the third piece. Serve!

**Nutritional Info:** Calories: 380; Fat: 22g; Carbs: 25.6g; Protein: 19g; Fiber: 3.9g

**Brazilian Fish Stew**

Time to prepare: 10 minutes
Time to cook: 19 minutes
Servings: 4

**Ingredients:**

- 1 to 1 1/2 lb. of firm white fish
- 1 lime's juice & zest
- ½ teaspoon salt

For the Sauce:

- 4 garlic cloves, chopped
- 1 onion, diced
- 1 red bell pepper, chopped (if tolerated)
- 1 (14 oz.) can of coconut milk
- 1 1/2 cups of chopped tomatoes, no seeds & peeled
- 1 cup carrot, diced
- 1 cup chicken stock
- ½ cup chopped herbs
- 2 to 3 tablespoon olive oil
- 1 tablespoon tomato paste
- ½ teaspoon salt
- 1 teaspoon ground cumin

**Directions:**

1. Rub the fish with the lime juice, zest, and 1 tablespoon of salt.

2. Saute the onion and salt in a pan for 2 to 3 minutes. For 4 to 5 minutes, add the bell pepper, carrot, and garlic.

3. After adding the tomato paste, stock, and spices, simmer for 5 minutes. Cook

the fish for 4 to 6 minutes after adding the coconut milk and stirring thoroughly. Serve!

**Nutritional Info:** Calories 404; Fat 19.7g; Carbs 12.6g; Protein 44g; Fiber 1.2g

**Prawn & Vegetable Pasta**

Time to prepare: 10 minutes
Time to cook: 30 minutes
Servings: 4

**Ingredients:**

- 18 medium prawns
- 6 oz of refined pasta, cooked & drained
- 1 large zucchini, peeled, seeded & spiralized
- 2 cups of baby spinach
- 1 1/2 cups of cherry tomatoes, peeled, halved & seeded
- ½ cup of fresh basil, sliced
- 2 minced garlic cloves
- 3 tablespoon olive oil
- 1 teaspoon oregano
- Salt & pepper to taste

**Directions:**

1. In a pan, cook the oregano, olive oil, and garlic for one minute. Cook for 5 minutes after adding the tomatoes. Cook the spinach after adding it until it wilts.

2. Cook the prawns in 1 tablespoon oil for 1 to 2 minutes on one side in a separate pan. Turn off the heat.

3. Include the basil, pasta, tomatoes, and zucchini noodles. Toss for 2 minutes. Serve it with prawns after seasoning it with salt and pepper.

**Nutritional Info:** Calories 246; Fat 5g; Carbs 14g; Protein 10g; Fiber 3g

**Turkey with Rosemary**

Time to prepare: 15 minutes
Time to cook: 10 minutes

Servings: 2

**Ingredients:**

- 1 lb. boneless, skinless turkey breasts, cut into bite-size pieces
- 2 minced garlic cloves
- 1/2 chopped onion
- 2 tablespoon extra-virgin olive oil
- 1 tablespoon chopped fresh rosemary leaves
- 1/4 teaspoon sea salt
- A pinch of freshly ground black pepper

**Directions:**

1. In a nonstick skillet or pan, heat the olive oil over medium-high heat.
2. Include the turkey, onion, rosemary, salt, and pepper. Cook the vegetables and turkey until they are both tender. Cook the turkey for an additional 30 seconds after adding it.

**Nutritional Info:** Calories: 413; Fat: 17g; Carbs: 6.8g; Protein: 54g; Fiber: 1.6g

### Grilled Salmon Steaks

Time to prepare: 5 minutes
Time to cook: 10 minutes
Servings: 2

**Ingredients:**

- 1 teaspoon olive oil
- 2 salmon steaks
- 2 tablespoon soy sauce

**Directions:**

1. Preheat the grill and oil the grate.
2. Brush the sauce over the fish fillets and cook them for 5 minutes on each side. Serve!

**Nutritional Info:** Calories 295; Fat 17g; Carbs 7g; Protein 31g; Fiber 0g

### Fiesta Chicken Tacos

Time to prepare: 10 minutes
Time to cook: 6 minutes

Servings: 8

**Ingredients:**

- 1 lb. chicken breast, skinless & boneless, cut into thin strips
- 8 well-tolerated corn tortillas, heated
- 1 cup of each sliced red bell pepper & red onion (if tolerated)
- 1 cup mixed salad greens
- 1 tablespoon olive oil
- ½ teaspoon ground cumin
- ¼ teaspoon salt

**Directions:**

1. Cumin is used to season the chicken. For three minutes, sauté in hot oil in a pan. Dispatch it on a plate.
2. Cook the onion and bell pepper for three minutes in one tablespoon of oil. Salt the chicken before adding it back to the pan.
3. Fill each tortilla with 2 tablespoons of mixed greens and the chicken mixture. Secure and serve with a roll.

**Nutritional Info:** Calories 320; Fat 6.4g; Carbs 36.1g; Protein 30.3g; Fiber 3.8g

### Shrimp Scampi Pizza

Time to prepare: 10 minutes
Time to cook: 20 minutes
Servings: 8

**Ingredients:**

- 1 (13.8 oz) pack of refined pizza dough
- 1 lb. peeled shrimp, cooked & sliced
- 2 cups shredded mozzarella
- 1 tablespoon cornmeal
- 1/2 cup ricotta cheese
- 6 cloves of roasted garlic
- 1 tablespoon dried basil
- Cooking spray

**Directions:**

1. Chicken is seasoned with cumin. In a pan, sauté for three minutes in hot oil. Put

it out on a plate. 2. In one tablespoon of oil, sauté the onion and bell pepper for three minutes. Before returning the chicken to the pan, season it with salt. 3. Place the chicken mixture and 2 tablespoons of mixed greens inside each tortilla. Serve with a roll after securing.

**Nutritional Info:** Calories 175; Fat 5g; Carbs 18.7g; Protein 14g; Fiber 1g

## Duck with Pear

Time to prepare: 10 minutes
Time to cook: 60 minutes
Servings: 2-3
**Ingredients:**

- 2 organic duck breasts
- 1 cup canned pear
- ¼ cup coconut oil
- 2 tablespoon garlic minced (if tolerated)
- ¼ cup honey
- 1 sprig of rosemary (if tolerated)
- 2 portions of lettuce leaves
- Himalayan salt to taste

**Directions:**

1. In your pan, warm the coconut oil, then add the rosemary, garlic, honey, and Himalayan salt. For a few minutes, cook.
2. In the interim, prepare a baking sheet and preheat the oven to 375°F.
3. Apply the mixture to the duck breasts and place them on the baking sheet. Roast for 60 to 75 minutes, or until thoroughly cooked. Serve!

**Nutritional Info:** Calories: 540; Fat: 23g; Carbs: 36g; Protein: 24g; Fiber: 1.2g

## Chicken Pasta with Zucchini

Time to prepare: 10 minutes
Time to cook: 6 minutes
Servings: 2
**Ingredients:**
- 1 tablespoon olive oil
- ½ cup red bell pepper, sliced
- 1 cup zucchini, peeled, seeded & sliced
- 2 cups cooked pasta, any shape
- 5 oz cooked chicken breast, sliced into strips
- 3 tablespoon low-sodium Italian dressing (if tolerated)

**Directions:**
1. In a nonstick skillet over medium heat, cook the peppers and zucchini until they are tender-crisp. Put on a dish.
2. Heat the cooked pasta and chicken strips separately in microwave-safe containers.
3. Combine the pasta and Italian dressing in a large mixing bowl. Before serving, top it with chicken strips and sautéed vegetables.
**Nutritional Info:** Calories: 400; Fat: 11g; Carbs: 45g; Protein: 30g; Fiber: 1.8g

## Chicken and Gnocchi Dumplings

Time to prepare: 20 minutes
Time to cook: 60 minutes
Servings: 10
**Ingredients:**
- 6-8 lb. chicken breast
- 1-lb store-bought gnocchi
- 6 cups reduced-sodium chicken stock
- ½ cup finely diced fresh carrots
- ½ cup finely diced fresh onions
- ½ cup of finely diced fresh celery
- ¼ cup fresh parsley, chopped
- ¼ cup olive oil
- 1 tablespoon low sodium chicken bouillon
- 1 teaspoon each of Italian seasoning & black pepper

**Directions:**
1. Set the stockpot over a high heat source and add the oil. In a hot skillet, cook the chicken until golden brown on all sides.
2. Add the celery, carrots, and onions, and then simmer the mixture with chicken stock for 20 to 30 minutes over high heat.
3. Reduce the heat to low and stir in the Italian seasoning, black pepper, and chicken bouillon. After adding the gnocchi, cook for 15 minutes while stirring frequently.
4. Add parsley to the dish and serve.
**Nutritional Info:** Calories: 362; Fat: 10g; Carbs: 38g; Protein: 28g; Fiber: 3.6g

## Crunchy Lemon Herbed Chicken

Time to prepare: 10 minutes
Time to cook: 10-15 minutes
Servings: 4
**Ingredients:**
- 4 tablespoon unsalted non-dairy butter (half chilled), divided
- 1 tablespoon fresh chopped thyme
- ½ cup Japanese bread crumbs
- 1 egg yolk
- 1 tablespoon + 3 teaspoon water
- 6 (2-oz) chicken tenders, pounded
- ½ cup cooked rice
- ¼ cup lemon juice, + the zest of 1 lemon
- 1 tablespoon fresh chopped basil

**Directions:**
1. In a small saucepan over medium-low heat, melt 2 tablespoons of butter. Toss the bread crumbs with half the herbs and

the lemon zest.

2. Combine 1 egg yolk and 1 tablespoon water in a mixing bowl.Apply the egg wash mixture to the chicken first, and then the herbed-breadcrumb mixture.

3. Melt the butter in a sauté pan over medium heat and add the breaded chicken.Cook the chicken for two to three minutes on each side. Before cutting it, let it cool.

4. In the same pan, combine the water, additional herbs, and lemon juice. Simmer the mixture gently.

5. Turn off the heat and whisk briskly before adding the remaining cooled butter.

6. Arrange the sliced chicken on a plate, top with sauce, and add the remaining herbs as a garnish.

**Nutritional Info:** Calories: 281; Fat: 20g; Carbs: 7g; Protein: 19g; Fiber: 4.3g

## Chicken with Garlic Yogurt Sauce

Time to prepare: 20 minutes
Time to cook: 1 hour
Servings: 4
**Ingredients:**
- 4 chicken thighs
- 1 teaspoon ground coriander
- 1 teaspoon lemon zest
- 1 lemon quartered, seeded
- ½ cup extra virgin olive oil
- ½ cup non-dairy yogurt
- 2 Spanish onions, cut into 1" wedges (if tolerated)
- 2 garlic heads, halved crosswise
- 2 garlic cloves
- 1 teaspoon lime zest
- freshly ground black pepper, to taste
- Water, as needed

**Directions:**
1. Preheat the oven to 325 F. Place the chicken thighs, onions, half-garlic cloves, and lemon quarters in a baking dish.
2. Drizzle them with oil, sprinkle salt and

pepper on top, and then dust them in flour. Roasting takes 50 minutes in the oven at 350 degrees.

3. In the meantime, grate one garlic clove and combine it with yogurt, pepper, and a little water to thin out the sauce. Except for the chicken thighs, remove the pan and put it aside.

4. Set the oven to 400°F and bake the chicken thighs for 10 minutes or until they are crisp.

5. In a bowl, mix the pan drippings with the lemon, lime, and pepper zests. Serve the baked chicken thighs after applying this mixture to them.

**Nutritional Info:** Calories: 413; Fat: 29.7g; Carbs: 9.3g; Protein: 26.7g; Fiber: 3.7g

## Turkey Meatballs with Apple Jelly

Time to prepare: 15 minutes
Time to cook: 21 minutes
Servings: 45 meatballs
**Ingredients:**
- 1 lb. lean ground turkey
- ½ cup unseasoned bread crumbs
- ¼ cup minced bell pepper
- ¼ cup minced onion
- ½ cup apple jelly
- 1 egg white
- 2 teaspoon Italian seasoning

**Directions:**
1. To 400°F, preheat the oven.
2. Combine all the ingredients—except the jelly—in a big bowl. the mixture into 45 meatballs.
3. Place your baking sheet with the meatballs on it, and bake for about 20 minutes, or until thoroughly cooked.
4. To liquefy the jelly, microwave it for roughly one minute. Put the meatballs and jelly in a serving dish.

**Nutritional Info:** Calories: 68; Fat: 3.1g; Carbs: 3.7g; Protein: 5.7g; Fiber: 4.1g

## Roasted Chicken with Mushroom Salad

Time to prepare: 10 minutes
Time to cook: 18 minutes
Servings: 2

**Ingredients:**
- 2 chicken breasts
- ½ teaspoon thyme
- 1 cup assorted wild mushrooms
- 4 tablespoon olive oil
- 2 tablespoon balsamic vinegar
- ½ cup shallots
- Black peppercorns to taste

**Directions:**

1. Add olive oil after seasoning the chicken with black pepper and thyme.
2. Set the oven to 350 degrees Fahrenheit, bake the chicken for 15 minutes, and check to make sure the inside is no longer pink.
3. Within 3 minutes, brown the mushrooms and shallots in your skillet with the oil. Fresh thyme is used as seasoning, and balsamic vinegar is added.
4. Slice your chicken and add warm mushrooms to the plate.

**Nutritional Info:** Calories: 340; Fat: 21g; Carbs: 6g; Protein: 31g; Fiber: 4.6g

## Ricotta and Herb Stuffed Chicken

Time to prepare: 15 minutes
Time to cook: 40 minutes
Servings: 4

**Ingredients:**
- 2 (6 oz each) large chicken breasts, boneless & skinless
- 1 garlic clove
- 1 egg
- ¼ cup chopped herbs
- 1 tablespoon extra virgin olive oil
- 1 1/2 cup ricotta
- ¼ teaspoon black pepper

**Directions:**

1. In a pan with olive oil, quickly sauté the garlic.
2. In a mixing bowl, combine the ricotta, eggs, garlic, and herbs.
3. Make a slit in the chicken breast's fattest side, then stuff it with the prepared mixture.
4. After the pan has heated up, brown the chicken in it for nine minutes. Add your baking sheet to it.
5. Bake the chicken for 20 to 30 minutes in a 350°F oven. Serve!

**Nutritional Info:** Calories: 277; Fat: 10g; Carbs: 5g; Protein: 32g; Fiber: 1.4g

## Chicken with Bell Peppers

Time to prepare: 10 minutes
Time to cook: 0 minutes
Servings: 6

**Ingredients:**
- 3 tablespoon olive oil, divided
- 1 lb. chicken breasts, boneless & skinless, cut thinly
- 3 large bell peppers, seeded & sliced
- 1 teaspoon dried oregano, crushed
- ¼ teaspoon garlic powder
- ¼ teaspoon ground cumin
- ¼ cup chicken bone broth
- sea salt & ground black pepper to taste

**Directions:**

1. In a skillet set over medium-high heat, heat 1 tablespoon of oil. Cook the bell peppers for about 4 minutes. Transfer the pepper mixture to a plate using a slotted spoon.
2. Cook the chicken in the remaining oil in the same skillet over medium-high heat for about 8 minutes, stirring frequently.
3. Add the thyme, spices, salt, and black pepper. Allow the broth to boil. Stir in the pepper mixture after adding it.
4. Adjust the heat to medium and cook, stirring occasionally, for about 3 minutes. Serve right away.

**Nutritional Info:** Calories 226; Fat 12.8g; Carbs 4.8g; Protein 22.9g; Fiber 0.9g

## Yummy Chicken Penne

Time to prepare: 10 minutes
Time to cook: 8 minutes
Servings: 4

**Ingredients:**
- 1 lb. raw chicken breast, sliced into 3" x 1" inch strips
- 2 cups refined penne pasta, cooked & drained
- 24 cherry tomatoes, peeled, seeded & halved
- 3 green onions cut into cubes
- ¼ cup chopped fresh basil
- 2 tablespoon cottage cheese
- 2 cloves garlic, minced
- 2 tablespoon olive oil, divided

**Directions:**

1. In a large nonstick skillet, heat 1 tablespoon of olive oil over medium-high heat. Cook the chicken strips for 2 to 3 minutes after adding them.

Pour the remaining oil in after adjusting the heat to medium. Once the chicken is fully cooked, add the tomatoes and garlic and cook for 3 to 4 minutes, or until the tomatoes burst.

3. After the green onions and cooked penne are added, cook for one minute.

4. In a dish, combine cottage cheese and basil. Serve this mixture on top of the spaghetti.

**Nutritional Info:** Calories: 392, Carbs: 39 g, Protein: 34 g, Fat: 10 g, Fiber: 2.5 g

## Moroccan Chicken

Time to prepare: 10 minutes + marinating time
Time to cook: 40 minutes
Servings: 6

**Ingredients:**

- 6 chicken breasts or thighs, bone-in, no skin
- 1 cup honey
- ½ teaspoon ground cumin
- ¼ teaspoon onion powder
- ¼ teaspoon cinnamon
- 1 teaspoon olive oil
- 2 tablespoon lemon juice
- ½ teaspoon lemon zest
- 3 cloves garlic, crushed

**Directions:**

1. Combine all the ingredients and use this mixture to marinate the chicken. Place in the refrigerator for up to 24 hours, turning occasionally.

2. Lay the chicken, bone-side down, on a baking sheet that has been lined with foil. On top, add the remaining marinade.

3. Preheat the oven to 400°F and bake the food for 30 to 40 minutes, or until thoroughly cooked.

**Nutritional Info:** Calories: 196; Fat: 3g; Carbs: 16g; Protein: 26g; Fiber: 1.4g

## Ground Turkey Skillet with Vegetables

Time to prepare: 15 minutes
Time to cook: 17 minutes
Servings: 3

**Ingredients:**
- 1 lb. ground turkey
- 3 radishes, chopped
- 1 large carrot, peeled & chopped
- 3 stalks of green onion, chopped
- 3 tablespoon coconut aminos
- 2 tablespoon avocado oil
- ½ teaspoon ground turmeric
- ½ teaspoon sea salt

**Directions:**

1. In a large cast-iron pan over medium-high heat, warm the avocado oil.

2. Arrange and compact the ground turkey into a single layer. The turkey should be golden brown after 2 to 3 minutes of browning it without touching

it.

3. Brown the meat on the other side for a further 2 minutes. It should be broken up, salted, and spiced.

4. Add the veggies to the skillet and give them a good toss. Cook the veggies covered for 5 to 10 minutes, or until they are tender.

5. After cooking for one to two minutes, add the coconut aminos. Stir thoroughly, then season to taste with more sea salt and coconut aminos. Serve!

**Nutritional Info:** Calories: 346; Fat: 21g; Carbs: 9g; Protein: 32g; Fiber: 4.2g

### Chicken & Potato Bake

Time to prepare: 15 minutes + marinating time
Time to cook: 48 minutes
Servings: 4

**Ingredients:**

- 4 (4-oz.) skinless chicken thighs
- 8 baby potatoes, peeled & halved
- 1 cup fresh lemon juice
- 3 tablespoon olive oil, divided
- 1 teaspoon dried parsley
- 1 teaspoon dried oregano
- Salt to taste

**Directions:**

1. In a large bowl, combine the salt, dried herbs, 2 tablespoons of oil, and lemon juice. In a  bowl, set aside half of the marinade.

2. In the remaining marinade dish, add the chicken thighs and well combine. Turn the chicken thighs every so often while covering and chilling them overnight.

3. Set the oven's temperature to 430°F.

4. Heat the remaining oil in a large oven-safe pan over medium-high heat. Sear the chicken thighs for 4 minutes on each side.

5. Remove the extra fat from the pan with a spoon, leaving approximately 1 tablespoon behind. Gently mix the potatoes with the marinade that has been saved.

6. Place your covered skillet in the oven and bake for about 35 minutes. The oven should be set to broil.

7. Take off the skillet's top, then broil the food for 5 to 10 minutes, or until the chicken and potatoes are browned and crispy. Let it cool before serving.

**Nutritional Info:** Calories: 395; Fat: 15.3g; Carbs: 40g; Protein: 25.6g; Fiber: 2.9g

### Chicken & Spinach Stew

Time to prepare: 15 minutes
Time to cook: 25 minutes
Servings: 8

**Ingredients:**

- 6 (4-oz.) chicken thighs, boneless, skinless, trimmed & cut into 1-inch pieces
- 4 tomatoes, peeled, seeded & chopped
- 4 cups fresh spinach, chopped
- 2 cups homemade chicken broth
- 2 tablespoon olive oil
- Salt & ground black pepper to taste

**Directions:**

1. In a large, heavy-bottomed pan, heat the oil over medium heat. Cook the chicken for 4 to 5 minutes.

2. Include the tomatoes, broth, salt, and black pepper. Simmer gently. Reduce to a low heat, cover, and leave to cook for ten to fifteen minutes.

3. Add the spinach and stir. Cook for 4-5 minutes. Serve warm.

**Nutritional Info:** Calories: 216; Fat: 10.3g; Carbs: 3.2g; Protein: 26.8g; Fiber: 1.1g

### Chicken & Asparagus Stew

Time to prepare: 10 minutes
Time to cook: 20 minutes
Servings: 6

**Ingredients:**

- 1 lb. chicken breasts, skinless & boneless, cubed
- 3 cups asparagus tips
- 2 cups homemade chicken broth
- 1 tablespoon olive oil
- Salt & ground black pepper to taste

**Directions:**

1. Heat the oil in your pan over medium heat before adding the chicken and cooking it for about 4-5 minutes. Let the broth boil after adding it.

2. Adjust the heat to low and cook for 8 to 10 minutes. Add the asparagus, season with salt and pepper, and cook for about 4-5 minutes, depending on how done you like your asparagus. Serve warm.

**Nutritional Info:** Calories: 157; Fat: 5.5g; Carbs: 4.3g; Protein: 21.5g; Fiber: 1.9g

### Chicken & Potato Curry

Time to prepare: 15 minutes
Time to cook: 30 minutes
Servings: 6

**Ingredients:**

- 4 (4-oz.) chicken breasts, boneless & skinless, cubed
- 1 lb. potato, peeled & cubed
- 2 tomatoes, peeled, seeded & chopped
- 2 cups homemade chicken broth
- 2 tablespoon olive oil
- Salt & ground black pepper to taste

**Directions:**

1. Add the chicken pieces, salt, and black pepper to the oil in your large sauté pan and stir for about 4 minutes.

2. Transfer the chicken onto a dish using a slotted spoon.

3. Add the tomatoes to the same pan and simmer for two to three minutes. For two to three minutes after adding the potatoes, let them cook.

4. Bring the stock and chicken to a boil. Cook for 15 to 20 minutes at medium-low heat. Serve immediately with the salt and black pepper.

**Nutritional Info:** Calories: 262; Fat: 10.9g; Carbs: 15.1g; Protein: 25.4g; Fiber: 2.1g

### Ground Turkey with Tomato Sauce

Time to prepare: 15 minutes
Time to cook: 39 minutes
Servings: 8

**Ingredients:**

- 2 lb. lean ground turkey
- 3 cups tomatoes, peeled, seeded & chopped finely
- 2 cups homemade chicken broth
- 2 oz sugar-free tomato paste
- 2 tablespoon olive oil
- Salt & ground black pepper to taste

**Directions:**

1. Place the turkey in the big skillet, add the oil, and cook for about 4-5 minutes.

2. Add the tomato paste and stir in the tomatoes; simmer for 3–4 minutes. Let the broth boil after adding it.

3. Lower the heat to a simmering point and cover the pot for approximately 30 minutes. Serve immediately after adding the salt and pepper.

**Nutritional Info:** Calories: 220; Fat: 12.1g; Carbs: 4.2g; Protein: 24.4g; Fiber: 1.1g

### Ground Turkey with Asparagus

Time to prepare: 10 minutes
Time to cook: 20 minutes
Servings: 8

**Ingredients:**

- 1¾ lb. lean ground turkey
- 4 cups asparagus tips
- ¼ cup water
- 2 tablespoon fresh parsley, chopped
- 1 tablespoon olive oil
- Salt & ground black pepper to taste

**Directions:**

1. Heat the oil in a large nonstick pan over medium heat. Add the turkey and cook for

8 to 10 minutes, or until browned.

2. Cook the asparagus for about 5 to 6 minutes after adding the water. Add the parsley, salt, and black pepper, and cook for 3 to 4 minutes while constantly stirring. Serve warm.

**Nutritional Info:** Calories: 187; Fat: 8.9g; Carbs: 4.1g; Protein: 22.5g; Fiber: 1.9g

## Turkey & Veggies Bake

Time to prepare: 15 minutes
Time to cook: 60 minutes
Servings: 6
**Ingredients:**

- 1 lb. lean ground turkey
- 2 large zucchinis, peeled, seeded & sliced
- 2 medium tomatoes, peeled, seeded & sliced
- 2 cups low-fat cottage cheese, shredded
- 1 cup sugar-free tomato sauce
- ½ cup low-fat cheddar cheese, shredded
- 1 egg yolk
- 1 tablespoon fresh rosemary, minced
- Salt & ground black pepper to taste

**Directions:**

1. Preheat your oven to 500°F and oil a large roasting pan.

2. Arrange the tomato and zucchini slices in the roasting pan that has been prepared and coat with cooking spray.

3. Remove from the oven after 10 to 12 minutes and set aside.Set your oven to 350 degrees.

4. In the meantime, brown the turkey in a nonstick skillet over medium-high heat for approximately 8 to 10 minutes. Cook for two to three minutes after adding tomato sauce.

5. Take the turkey mixture out and put it in a 13- by 9-inch shallow baking dish.

6. Add the other ingredients to your bowl and stir to incorporate. The roasted veggies should be placed on top of the turkey mixture, followed by the cheese combination.

7. Bake for 35 minutes, then remove and let stand for 5 to 10 minutes. Let it cool before serving.

**Nutritional Info:** Calories: 252; Fat: 11.1g; Carbs: 9.3g; Protein: 29.7g; Fiber: 2g

## Turkey Meatloaf

Time to prepare: 15 minutes
Time to cook: 40 minutes
Servings: 8
**Ingredients:**
For the Meatloaf:

- 2 lb. lean ground turkey
- 1 egg
- 1 cup low-fat cheddar cheese, shredded
- 2 oz sugar-free tomato sauce
- Salt to taste

For Topping:

- 2 oz sugar-free tomato sauce
- ½ cup low-fat cheddar cheese, shredded

**Directions:**

1. Preheat your oven to 400 degrees Fahrenheit and grease a 9- by 13-inch casserole dish.

2. Place all the meatloaf ingredients in a bowl and stir to thoroughly combine. Spread the mixture evenly across the bottom of the casserole dish you have prepared.

3. Evenly spread tomato sauce over the meatloaf's top and top with cheese.

4. Bake for 40 minutes, then serve after it has cooled.

**Nutritional Info:** Calories: 259; Fat: 15.7g; Carbs: 1.1g; Protein: 28.4g; Fiber: 0.8g

## Turkey Stuffed Bell Peppers

Time to prepare: 15 minutes

Time to cook: 31 minutes
Servings: 5
**Ingredients:**
- 1 lb. lean ground turkey
- 5 large bell peppers, tops & seeds removed
- 1 large zucchini, peeled, seeded & chopped
- 1 tablespoon olive oil
- ½ teaspoon dried oregano
- ½ teaspoon dried thyme
- 3 tablespoon tomato paste
- Salt & ground black pepper to taste

**Directions:**
1. Preheat your oven to 350 degrees Fahrenheit, and grease a small baking dish.
2. Boil the bell peppers for four to five minutes in a big pot of water. Remove and place cut side down on a piece of paper towel.
3. In the meantime, in a big nonstick skillet, heat the olive oil over medium heat. For about 8 to 10 minutes, cook the ground turkey with the oregano, salt, and pepper.
4. Continue to cook the zucchini for two to three minutes. The beef mixture's juices should be removed and drained.
5. Add the tomato paste and combine by stirring. Place the bell peppers cut side up in the baking dish that has been prepared.
6. Evenly tuck the turkey mixture into each bell pepper. Serve hot after 15 minutes of baking.

**Nutritional Info:** Calories: 206; Fat: 9.7g; Carbs: 12.3g; Protein: 19.9g; Fiber: 2g

## Oregano Chicken Breast

Time to prepare: 10 minutes
Time to cook: 19 minutes
Servings: 6
**Ingredients:**
- 4 (7-oz.) boneless, skinless chicken breasts
- 1 tablespoon olive oil
- 1 teaspoon dried oregano
- Salt & ground black pepper to taste

**Directions:**
1. Preheat the oven to 425 degrees Fahrenheit and line a baking pan with parchment paper. Each chicken breast should be lightly pounded with a meat mallet.
2. In a bowl, combine the oil, oregano, salt, and black pepper. Add the chicken breasts and generously brush them with the oil mixture.
3. Place the chicken breasts in a single layer on the baking dish that has been prepared.
4. After baking the chicken breasts for 16 minutes, turn on the broiler for a couple of minutes. Slice it after cooling, then serve!

**Nutritional Info:** Calories: 272; Fat: 12.2g; Carbs: 0.2g; Protein: 38.3g; Fiber: 0.1g

## Zingy Chicken Breasts

Time to prepare: 10 minutes + marinating time
Time to cook: 20 minutes
Servings: 4
**Ingredients:**
- 4 (4-oz.) boneless, skinless chicken breasts
- 2 tablespoon olive oil
- 2 tablespoon fresh lime juice
- Salt & ground black pepper to taste

**Directions:**
1. Place all the ingredients in a large Ziploc bag and seal it. Shake the bag to thoroughly coat the chicken in the marinade.
2. Marinate in the refrigerator for 20 to 60 minutes. Grease the grill grate and heat the grill to a medium-high temperature.
3. Put the chicken breasts on the grill and

cook them for about 10 minutes on each side. Serve warm.

**Nutritional Info:** Calories: 276; Fat: 15.4g; Carbs: 0.1g; Protein: 32.8g; Fiber: 0g

## Sweet & Sour Chicken Breasts

Time to prepare: 10 minutes
Time to cook: 10 minutes
Servings: 4
**Ingredients:**
- 4 (4-oz.) chicken breast halves, boneless & skinless, pounded into the ½-inch thickness
- 1-2 tablespoon fresh cilantro, chopped
- 2 tablespoon fresh lime juice
- 1 tablespoon honey

**Directions:**
1. Turn on the oven's broiler and grease a broiler pan.
2. In a dish, combine the cilantro, lime juice, and honey. Apply a liberal amount of the honey mixture to each chicken breast.
3. Place the chicken breast in a single layer on the broiler pan that has been prepared, and broil for approximately 5 minutes per side. Serve warm.

**Nutritional Info:** Calories: 146; Fat: 2.8g; Carbs: 4.4g; Protein: 24.1g; Fiber: 0g

## Feta Stuffed Chicken Breasts

Time to prepare: 10 minutes
Time to cook: 17 minutes
Servings: 4
**Ingredients:**
- 4 (5-oz.) skinless, boneless chicken breasts, pounded into 1/8-inch thickness
- 4 oz. low-fat feta cheese, crumbled
- 4 tablespoon olive oil, divided
- 2 tablespoon fresh oregano, minced
- ½ teaspoon lemon zest, grated
- Salt & ground black pepper to taste

**Directions:**

1. Set the oven to 450°F.
2. Season the chicken breasts with salt and black pepper after brushing them with 2 tablespoons of oil. The chicken breasts should be arranged on a flat surface.
3. Place a thin layer of feta on top of each chicken breast, then garnish with oregano and lemon zest. To tightly seal the filling, roll each breast like a jelly roll.
4. Tie each roll at intervals of 1 inch with one piece of kitchen twine.
5. Cook the chicken rolls for 10 minutes, or until they are browned on both sides, in the remaining oil in the pan over medium heat. Take the chicken rolls' cooking pan from the stove.
6. Arrange the rolls in a single layer in a baking dish. Baking takes around 5-7 minutes. Serve warm.

**Nutritional Info:** Calories: 379; Fat: 21.3g; Carbs: 2.7g; Protein: 35.9g; Fiber: 1.2g

## Parmesan Tomato Chicken

Time to prepare: 10 minutes
Time to cook: 13 minutes
Servings: 4
**Ingredients:**
- 4 (4-oz.) boneless, skinless chicken breasts
- 1 cup tomato sauce
- ½ cup part-skim mozzarella cheese, shredded
- 1 tablespoon olive oil
- 1 teaspoon dried thyme
- 1 teaspoon dried parsley
- ½ teaspoon dried oregano
- Salt & ground black pepper to taste

**Directions:**
1. Set the oven's broiler to medium heat.
2. Combine the tomato sauce and thyme in a bowl. Place aside.

3. In a small dish, combine the oil, herbs, salt, and black pepper. Apply the oil mixture to each chicken fillet on both sides.

4. Cook the chicken breasts for approximately 3 to 4 minutes on each side in a large, heavy, oven-safe pan that has been heated over high heat.

5. Distribute the tomato sauce equally over and around the chicken. Each chicken breast should have 2 tablespoons of the mozzarella on it.

6. Place your pan in the oven and turn on the broiler for 3 to 5 minutes, or until the cheese is melted. Serve warm.

**Nutritional Info:** Calories: 273; Fat: 12.7g; Carbs: 3.7g; Protein: 34.7g; Fiber: 1.1g

## Lemony Chicken Thighs

Time to prepare: 10 minutes + marinating time
Time to cook: 16 minutes
Servings: 6
**Ingredients:**
- 1½ lb. skinless, boneless chicken thighs
- 2 tablespoon olive oil, divided
- 1 tablespoon fresh lemon juice
- 1 tablespoon lemon zest, grated
- 2 teaspoon dried oregano
- 1 teaspoon dried thyme
- Salt & ground black pepper to taste

**Directions:**
1. Set the oven to 420°F.
2. In a bowl, add 1 tablespoon olive oil, lemon juice, zest, dried herbs, salt, and black pepper.
3. Place the chicken thighs in the basin and cover with the oil mixture. Marinate in the refrigerator for at least 25 to 30 minutes.
4. Heat the remaining oil in an oven-safe pan over medium-high heat, then sear the chicken thighs for two to three minutes

on each side.
5. Put the pan in the oven right away and bake for 10 minutes. Serve warm.
**Nutritional Info:** Calories: 185; Fat: 8.8g; Carbs: 0.7.1g; Protein: 25.4g; Fiber: 0.3g

## Maple-Glazed Chicken Thighs

Time to prepare: 15 minutes + marinating time
Time to cook: 25 minutes
Servings: 5
**Ingredients:**
- 5 (4-oz.) skinless chicken thighs
- 2 tablespoon fresh lime juice
- 2 tablespoon maple syrup
- 2 tablespoon olive oil
- Salt & ground black pepper to taste

**Directions:**
1. In a bowl, thoroughly mix all the toppings, except the chicken thighs and sesame seeds.
2. Place the marinade and chicken thighs in a large plastic zipper bag. to thoroughly coat, seal, and shake the bag. Turn the bag over twice in the refrigerator within an hour.
3. Set the oven to 425°F. The chicken should be removed, and any extra marinade should be saved.
4. Spread some of the prepared marinade over the chicken thighs and arrange them in a single layer in a 9 x 13-inch baking dish.
5. Bake for 25 minutes, brushing with a little of the remaining marinade every 10 minutes. Serve warm.

**Nutritional Info:** Calories: 285; Fat: 14g; Carbs: 5.4g; Protein: 32.8g; Fiber: 0g

## Chicken In Orange Sauce

Time to prepare: 15 minutes + marinating time
Time to cook: 17 minutes
Servings: 6
**Ingredients:**

- 2 lb. skinless, bone-in chicken thighs
- ½ cup fresh orange juice
- 1 tablespoon apple cider vinegar
- Salt & ground black pepper to taste

**Directions:**

1. In a large dish, combine all the ingredients with the exception of the chicken thighs. Add the chicken thighs and thoroughly brush them with the marinade.

2. Within two hours, cover and marinate in the refrigerator. With the marinade still in the bowl, remove the chicken thighs.

3. Place your large nonstick pan on the stovetop and heat it to medium-high heat. Cook the chicken for about 5 to 6 minutes, or until it turns golden brown.

4. After 3 minutes, flip the side and continue cooking. Let it boil before adding the marinade you saved.

5. Lower the heat to medium-low and cook the sauce, covered, for 6 to 8 minutes, or until it thickens. Serve warm.

**Nutritional Info:** Calories: 199; Fat: 5.4g; Carbs: 2.2g; Protein: 33.9g; Fiber: 0g|

## Tomato Sauce Glazed Chicken Thighs

Time to prepare: 10 minutes
Time to cook: 15 minutes
Servings: 4

**Ingredients:**

- 4 (4-oz.) skinless, boneless chicken thighs
- ½ cup sugar-free tomato sauce
- 2½ tablespoon apple cider vinegar
- 2 tablespoon fresh cilantro, minced
- 1 tablespoon olive oil
- Salt & ground black pepper to taste

**Directions:**

1. Combine all the ingredients in a glass baking dish—aside from the chicken thighs—thoroughly. Add the chicken thighs and generously coat with the mixture.

2. Marinate overnight in the refrigerator.

The large baking sheet should be lined with greased foil. Preheat the oven's broiler.

3. Take out the chicken thighs from the bowl and set aside the marinade. Place the chicken thighs in a single layer on the baking sheet that has been prepared, and broil for 5 minutes on each side.

4. In the meantime, add the reserved marinade to a small pan and cook for 8 to 10 minutes over medium heat. The glaze-topped chicken thighs should be served.

**Nutritional Info:** Calories: 187; Fat: 7.6g; Carbs: 2g; Protein: 25.7g; Fiber: 0.5g

## Chicken In Yogurt Sauce

Time to prepare: 10 minutes
Time to cook: 18 minutes
Servings: 6

**Ingredients:**

- 1½ lb. chicken breasts, cut into ¾-inch chunks
- 2 tomatoes, peeled, seeded & chopped finely
- 1 cup fat-free plain yogurt
- 2 tablespoon fresh cilantro, chopped
- 2 tablespoon olive oil
- Salt & ground black pepper to taste

**Directions:**

1. In a large skillet, heat the oil over medium-high heat. When the tomatoes are ready, crush them with the back of a spoon and cook for about 2–3 minutes.

2. Add the black pepper and salt to the chicken and cook for 4-5 minutes. Yogurt should be added and cooked for an additional 8 to 10 minutes while stirring occasionally. Add the cilantro, then serve hot.

**Nutritional Info:** Calories: 281; Fat: 13.2g; Carbs: 4.4g; Protein: 34.8g; Fiber: 0.5g

## Chicken With Spinach

Time to prepare: 10 minutes

Time to cook: 9 minutes
Servings: 6
**Ingredients:**
- 1 lb. chicken tenders
- 14 oz frozen spinach, thawed
- ¼ cup fat-free plain yogurt
- 2 tablespoon olive oil, divided
- Salt & ground black pepper to taste

**Directions:**
1. Heat 1 tablespoon of oil in a large skillet over medium-high heat. Add the chicken and season with salt and black pepper. Cook for about 2–3 minutes per side. Place the bowl with the chicken inside.
2. Cook the spinach for about a minute in the remaining oil in the same skillet over medium-low heat.
3. Combine the yogurt, salt, and black pepper after adding them. In an even layer, cover the bottom of the skillet with the spinach mixture.
4. Spread the spinach with a single layer of chicken. Cook for about 5 minutes at a low temperature under cover. Serve warm.

**Nutritional Info:** Calories: 214; Fat: 11.4g; Carbs: 3.2g; Protein: 25g; Fiber: 1.5g

## Chicken With Green Beans

Time to prepare: 10 minutes
Time to cook: 13 minutes
Servings: 6
**Ingredients:**
- 1 lb. chicken breasts, boneless & skinless, cut thinly
- 1 lb. canned green beans, drained
- ¼ cup homemade chicken broth
- 2 tablespoon olive oil
- Salt & ground black pepper to taste

**Directions:**
1. In your sauté pan, heat the oil over medium-high heat. Cook the chicken, stirring frequently, for about 4-5 minutes.
2. After adding the green beans, cook for 2 to 3 minutes. Boiling ensues after adding the broth, salt, and black pepper.
3. Adjust the heat to medium and cook, stirring occasionally, for about 3 to 5 minutes, or until all the liquid is absorbed. Serve right away.

**Nutritional Info:** Calories: 226; Fat: 12.4g; Carbs: 0.9g; Protein: 26.7g; Fiber: 0.4g

## Chicken With Pumpkin

Time to prepare: 10 minutes
Time to cook: 25 minutes
Servings: 4
**Ingredients:**
- 2 (6-oz.) chicken breasts, skinless, boneless, cut into bite-sized pieces
- 1 (2-lb.) pumpkin, peeled, seeded & cubed
- 2 cups chicken broth
- 2 tablespoon olive oil
- Salt, to taste

**Directions:**
1. In a large skillet, heat the oil over medium heat. Cook the chicken pieces for 4-5 minutes.
2. Add the broth and pumpkin and bring to a boil. Cook at the desired thickness under cover for 15 to 20 minutes. Serve hot and sprinkle with salt.

**Nutritional Info:** Calories: 226; Fat: 12.8g; Carbs: 4.8g; Protein: 22.9g; Fiber: 0.9g

# LEAN MEATS

## Simple Strip Steaks

Time to prepare: 10 minutes
Time to cook: 8 minutes
Servings: 2
**Ingredients:**
- 2 (4-oz.) strip steaks, trimmed
- 2 teaspoon olive oil
- Salt & ground black pepper to taste

**Directions:**
1. Heat the oil in a big, heavy-bottomed skillet over high heat. Add the steaks, season with salt and black pepper, and cook for 3 to 4 minutes on each side.
2. Place the steaks on a chopping board and let them sit there for approximately 5 minutes before cutting. Serve!
**Nutritional Info:** Calories: 261; Fat: 12.8g; Carbs: 0g; Protein: 34.4g; Fiber: 0g

## Herbed Flank Steak

Time to prepare: 10 minutes
Time to cook: 20 minutes
Servings: 6
**Ingredients:**
- 1½ lb. flank steak, trimmed
- ½ teaspoon dried thyme, crushed
- ½ teaspoon dried oregano, crushed
- Salt & ground black pepper to taste

**Directions:**
1. Combine the dried herbs and spices in a sizable bowl. Add the steaks and generously rub them with the mixture. Set aside for about 15 to 20 minutes.
2. Grease the grill grate and warm it to medium heat.
3. Place the steak on your grill, flipping it once after 18 to 20 minutes. Serve!
**Nutritional Info:** Calories: 221; Fat: 9.5g; Carbs: 0.1g; Protein: 31.6g; Fiber: 0.1g

## Parsley Flank Steak

Time to prepare: 5 minutes
Time to cook: 10 minutes
Servings: 4
**Ingredients:**
- 4 (6-oz.) flank steaks
- 2 tablespoon olive oil
- 2 tablespoon fresh parsley, minced
- Salt & ground black pepper to taste

**Directions:**
1. Heat the oil in a pan over medium-high heat. Add the steaks, season with salt and black pepper, and cook for 4-5 minutes per side.
2. Take the steaks out of the pan and let them rest for about 10 minutes before slicing. Serve!
**Nutritional Info:** Calories: 260; Fat: 14.1g; Carbs: 0.1g; Protein: 31.6g; Fiber: 0g

## Thyme Tenderloin Fillets

Time to prepare: 10 minutes
Time to cook: 15 minutes
Servings: 4
**Ingredients:**
- 4 (6-oz.) beef tenderloin fillets
- 2 tablespoon olive oil
- 1 tablespoon fresh thyme, chopped
- Salt & ground black pepper to taste

**Directions:**
1. Evenly season the beef fillets with salt and black pepper, then place in a separate bowl. Thyme should be sautéed for approximately a minute in oil heated over medium heat in a cast-iron sauté pan.
2. Add the fillets and cook them for 5-7 minutes on each side. Serve!

**Nutritional Info:** Calories: 275; Fat: 15.1g; Carbs: 0.3g; Protein: 32.9g; Fiber: 0.2g

## Rosemary Beef Tenderloin

Time to prepare: 10 minutes
Time to cook: 50 minutes
Servings: 4
**Ingredients:**

- 1 (2-lb.) beef tenderloin
- 1/2 tablespoon fresh rosemary, minced
- 1/2 tablespoon olive oil
- Salt & ground black pepper to taste

**Directions:**

1. Preheat your oven to 425 degrees Fahrenheit, then oil a big shallow roasting pan.
2. Put the roast in the roasting pan that has been prepared. Add oil after seasoning the roast with rosemary, salt, and black pepper.
3. The beef should be roasted for 45 to 50 minutes. The beef tenderloin should be taken out of the oven and left to rest on a cutting board for about 10 minutes. Serve!

**Nutritional Info:** Calories: 245; Fat: 11.6g; Carbs: 0.2g; Protein: 32.8g; Fiber: 0.1g

## Beef With Carrot

Time to prepare: 10 minutes
Time to cook: 15 minutes
Servings: 4
**Ingredients:**

- 1 lb. beef tenderloin, trimmed and cut into thin strips
- 3 large carrots, peeled and sliced
- ¼ cup homemade chicken broth
- 2 tablespoon olive oil
- 1 tablespoon fresh lemon juice

- Salt & ground black pepper to taste

**Directions:**

1. In a large nonstick skillet over high heat, heat the oil. Sear the beef strips for 4–5 minutes, or until fully cooked. Transfer the beef into a bowl using a slotted spoon.
2. Add the carrot to the same skillet and cook for three to five minutes.
3. Stirring occasionally, cook the cooked beef mixture for 3 to 5 minutes. Add the broth, lemon juice, salt, and black pepper. Serve warm.

**Nutritional Info:** Calories: 213; Fat: 11.7g; Carbs: 3.6g; Protein: 22.4g; Fiber: 0.g

## Beef With Zucchini

Time to prepare: 10 minutes
Time to cook: 15 minutes
Servings: 6
**Ingredients:**

- 16 oz sirloin steak, trimmed & cut into thin strips
- 4 cups zucchini, peeled, seeded & chopped
- ¼ cup homemade chicken broth
- 2 tablespoon olive oil, divided
- 2 tablespoon fresh lime juice
- Salt & ground black pepper to taste

**Directions:**

1. Sprinkle salt and black pepper on the steak slices.
2. Cook the steak slices in a large sauté pan with 1 tablespoon oil over medium heat for about 4-5 minutes, or until browned on all sides.
3. Sliding the steak slices onto a plate using a slotted spoon
4. In the same sauté pan, heat the remaining oil over medium heat and cook the zucchini for 4-5 minutes.
5. Add the broth, lime juice, and steak

slices that have been cooked. Cook for three to five minutes. Serve warm.

**Nutritional Info:** Calories: 195; Fat: 9.6g; Carbs: 2.6g; Protein: 24g; Fiber: 0.8g

## Beef & Zucchini Soup

Time to prepare: 10 minutes
Time to cook: 20 minutes
Servings: 6

**Ingredients:**
- 1 lb. cooked beef, sliced thinly
- 1 lb. zucchini, peeled, seeded & chopped
- 6 cups homemade beef broth
- ¼ cup fresh parsley, chopped
- 2 tablespoon fresh lemon juice
- Salt & ground black pepper to taste

**Directions:**
1. Bring broth, beef, and zucchini to a boil in a soup pan. Simmer for approximately 10 minutes after adjusting the heat to medium-low.
2. Cook for about 5 minutes after adding parsley, lemon juice, salt, and black pepper. Serve warm.

**Nutritional Info:** Calories: 193; Fat: 6.3g; Carbs: 3.7g; Protein: 28.8g; Fiber: 0.9g

## Beef & Carrot Stew

Time to prepare: 10 minutes
Time to cook: 55 minutes
Servings: 6

**Ingredients:**
- 1½ lb. beef stew meat, trimmed & cubed
- 3 carrots, peeled and sliced
- 4 cup homemade beef broth
- 1 cup tomato puree
- 1 tablespoon olive oil
- 1 teaspoon dried parsley
- Salt & ground black pepper to taste

**Directions:**

1. In a large bowl, combine the beef cubes, salt, and black pepper. Toss to evenly coat.
2. Cook the beef cubes in your large skillet over medium-high heat for about 4-5 minutes, or until browned.
3. Add the remaining ingredients and combine by stirring. Set the heat to high and allow it to boil.
4. Adjust the heat to low and simmer for 40 to 50 minutes with the lid on. Serve immediately after seasoning with salt and black pepper.

**Nutritional Info:** Calories: 285; Fat: 10.4g; Carbs: 7.4g; Protein: 38.5g; Fiber: 1.6g

## Beef & Tomato Curry

Time to prepare: 10 minutes
Time to cook: 21 minutes
Servings: 8

**Ingredients:**
- 2½ lb. beef chuck roast, trimmed & cubed
- 4 tomatoes, peeled, seeded & chopped finely
- 2 cups homemade chicken broth
- ¼ cup fresh cilantro, chopped
- 2 tablespoon olive oil
- Salt & ground black pepper to taste

**Directions:**
1. In a large skillet over low heat, heat the oil. Cook the tomatoes for 3 to 4 minutes, crushing them as they cook.
2. Add the broth and simmer gently while stirring from time to time. For about 4–5 minutes, simmer.
3. Add the beef and cook on medium heat until boiling. Set to low heat, cover, and cook for about two hours, stirring occasionally.
4. After adding the cilantro, season with salt and black pepper. Cook for 5 to 10 minutes. Serve warm.

**Nutritional Info:** Calories: 253; Fat: 11.9g; Carbs: 2.1g; Protein: 32.5g; Fiber: 0.6g

## Ground Beef with Mushrooms

Time to prepare: 10 minutes
Time to cook: 20 minutes
Servings: 4
**Ingredients:**
- 1 lb. lean ground beef
- 2 cups fresh mushrooms, sliced
- ¼ cup homemade chicken broth
- 2 tablespoon fresh basil
- 2 tablespoon olive oil
- 2 tablespoon fresh parsley, chopped
- 1 tablespoon fresh lemon juice

**Directions:**
1. In a sizable nonstick sauté pan that has been heated to medium-high heat, add the ground beef and cook, breaking up the chunks with a wooden spoon, for about 8 to 10 minutes.
2. Put the beef in a bowl with a slotted spoon.
3. Include the mushrooms and cook for 5 to 7 minutes in the same sauté pan. Bring to a boil after adding the cooked beef, basil, broth, and lemon juice.
4. Adjust the heat to medium-low and simmer for about three minutes. Add the parsley and serve right away.
**Nutritional Info:** Calories: 280; Fat: 13.2g; Carbs: 2.2g; Protein: 35g; Fiber: 0.6g

## Garlic Lime Pork Chops

Time to prepare: 10 minutes + marinating time
Time to cook: 10 minutes
Servings: 4
**Ingredients:**
- 4 (6 oz each) lean boneless pork chops

- 4 cloves garlic, crushed
- 1 teaspoon cumin
- Juice of ½ lime
- Zest of ½ lime
- Fresh black pepper to taste

**Directions:**
1. In a bowl, season the pork with all the herbs and spices, lime juice, zest, and garlic. 20 minutes of marinating
2. Place tin foil on top of the broiler pan. Broil the seasoned pork for 5 minutes on each side in the pan. Serve hot.
**Nutritional Info:** Calories 402; Fat 9.8g; Carbs 21.1g; Protein 44 g; Fiber 3.1g

## Lamb With Low-Fiber Pesto

Time to prepare: 10 minutes
Time to cook: 0 minutes
Servings: 4
**Ingredients:**
- 1 lb. organic lamb fillets, pounded
- 1 small carrot, peeled & chopped
- 1½ cups asparagus tips
- 1 cup canned green beans, halved
- 2 teaspoon olive oil

For the Low-Fiber Pesto:
- ½ cup basil leaves
- 3 tablespoon extra virgin olive oil
- 2 tablespoon apple cider vinegar
- 1 tablespoon soft cheddar
- ¼ teaspoon Himalayan salt

**Directions:**
1. The oven should be heated to 375°F.
2. In the meantime, puree all of the pesto ingredients in a blender until smooth. Place aside.
3. In a hot pan, sear the lamb fillets for a few minutes on each side. In a baking dish, combine the vegetables and the lamb fillets.
4. Wrap in foil and place in the oven for 25 to 30 minutes of baking. Remove and

spread pesto on top to create a crust. Serve!

**Nutritional Info:** Calories: 392; Fat: 31g; Carbs: 6g; Protein: 20.1g; Fiber: 2.2g

## Broiled Lamb Chops

Time to prepare: 10 minutes
Time to cook: 10 minutes
Servings: 4

**Ingredients:**
- 8 (around 4 oz) of lamb loin chops
- ¼ teaspoon black pepper
- ½ teaspoon salt
- 1 tablespoon minced garlic
- 2 tablespoon lemon juice
- 1 tablespoon dried oregano
- Cooking spray

**Directions:**
1. Preheat the broiler in your oven.
2. Combine the oregano, black pepper, salt, chopped garlic, and lemon juice in a large basin. Next, evenly massage it into the lamb chops on both sides.
3. Spray cooking spray on a broiler pan before adding the lamb chops, and then broil for 5 minutes on each side.

**Nutritional Info:** Calories 332; Fat 16g; Carbs 3g; Protein 46g; Fiber 0.3g

## Mustard Chops with Apricot-Basil Relish

Time to prepare: 10 minutes
Time to cook: 12 minutes
Servings: 4

**Ingredients:**
- 4 lean pork chops
- ¾ lb. fresh or canned apricots, stone removed, & fruit diced
- 3 tablespoon raspberry vinegar
- 1 teaspoon ground cardamom
- 2 tablespoon olive oil
- ¼ cup basil, finely shredded
- 1 shallot, diced small
- ½ cup mustard
- Pepper & salt to taste

**Directions:**
1. Salt and pepper are used to season the pork chops. Apply mustard to each pork chop's top and bottom. Fire up the grill to a medium-high temperature.
2. In a medium bowl, combine the cardamom, olive oil, vinegar, basil, shallot, and apricots. Mix well after tossing, then season with salt and pepper.
3. Cook the chops for 5 to 6 minutes on each side. Apply the mustard baste as you flip. Enjoy the apricot-basil relish with the pork chops.

**Nutritional Info:** Calories 488; Fat 25g; Carbs 22g; Protein 42g; Fiber 3g

## Beef Ragu

Time to prepare: 10 minutes
Time to cook: 10 minutes
Servings: 2

**Ingredients:**
- ¼ lb. ground beef
- ¼ cup packaged pesto
- 2 large zucchinis, peeled, seeded & cut into noodle strips
- 4 tablespoon fresh parsley, chopped
- 1 tablespoon olive oil
- 1 teaspoon salt

**Directions:**
1. In a pan over medium heat, heat the oil. Cook the ground beef for 5 minutes, or until it is well cooked. Get rid of extra fat.
2. Include the pesto sauce and add salt. Cook for three more minutes after adding the chopped parsley. Place aside.
3. Add the zucchini noodles to the same pot and simmer for 5 minutes. Add the cooked meat after turning off the heat. Mix thoroughly, then plate.

**Nutritional Info:** Calories 353; Fat 30g; Carbs 2g; Protein 19g; Fiber 0.7g

## Traditional Scotch Eggs

Time to prepare: 15 minutes
Time to cook: 8 minutes
Servings: 5

**Ingredients:**
- 1 ½ lb. ground pork
- 5 eggs, hardboiled & peeled
- 1 egg, beaten
- 1 garlic clove minced
- ½ teaspoon paprika powder

**Directions:**
1. In a mixing bowl, combine the beaten egg, ground pork, garlic, and paprika. To taste, add salt and pepper to the food.
2. Make five balls out of the meat mixture. With your hands, flatten each ball, then position an egg in the middle. Apply the meat mixture over the egg. Use the other balls in the same way.
3. Cook the ground pork in a nonstick pan over medium heat for 4 minutes on each side. Enjoy after serving.

**Nutritional Info:** Calories 481; Fat 33g; Carbs 0.7g; Protein 42g; Fiber 0.1g

## Stir-Fried Mushrooms Beef Strips

Time to prepare: 10 minutes
Time to cook: 23 minutes
Servings: 4

**Ingredients:**
- 4 (1 lb.) beef steaks, cut into strips
- 2 cups mushrooms, sliced
- ¼ cup water
- 2 cloves of garlic, minced
- 2 tablespoon olive oil
- ½ teaspoon salt

**Directions:**
1. In a skillet with hot oil, sauté the garlic until fragrant. For three minutes, stir in the beef strips until they are lightly golden.

2. Add water and season to taste with salt and pepper. 15 minutes should pass while it simmers with the lid closed.
3. Add the salt and the mushrooms. Cook for an additional five minutes. Enjoy after serving.

**Nutritional Info:** Calories 226; Fat 13g; Carbs 1.7; Protein 24g; Fiber 0.2g

## Grilled Steak with Fish Sauce

Time to prepare: 10 minutes + marinating time
Time to cook: 8 minutes
Servings: 4

Ingredients
- 1 lb. grass-fed beef skirt steak, trimmed and cut into 4-inch slices lengthwise
- 2 teaspoon fresh ginger root, grated
- 2 teaspoon fresh lime zest, grated
- ¼ cup of coconut sugar
- 2 teaspoon red boat fish sauce
- 2 tablespoon fresh lime juice
- ½ cup unsweetened coconut milk
- Salt, to taste

**Directions:**
1. Combine all the ingredients in a sizable, sealable bag, excluding the steak and salt. Add the meat and liberally cover with marinade.
2. Seal the steak's bag and place it in the fridge for 4 to 12 hours of marinating. Grease the grill grate and heat the grill to a high temperature.
3. Take the meat out of the marinade and throw it away. The steak should be well dried with a paper towel before being equally salted.
4. Cook the steak slices for 3 to 12 minutes on the grill. For the desired doneness, flip the side and cook for an additional 3–5 minutes. Slice, then dish.

**Nutritional Info:** Calories 297; Fat 15.7g; Carbs 15.8g; Protein 24.1g; Fiber 0.9g

## Flank Steak with Honey Sauce

Time to prepare: 10 minutes
Time to cook: 22 minutes
Servings: 3

**Ingredients:**

- 1 lb. grass-fed flank steak, cut into ¼-inch thick slices
- 2 tablespoon refined flour
- ½ cup + 1 tablespoon coconut oil
- 2 garlic cloves, minced
- 1 teaspoon ground ginger
- 1/3 cup raw honey
- ½ cup low-sodium beef broth
- ½ cup coconut aminos
- 3 scallions, chopped
- Pinch of red pepper flakes, crushed
- Salt & ground black pepper to taste

**Directions:**

1. In a bowl, combine the flour, salt, and black pepper. Spread the flour mixture evenly over the meat pieces. Shake off any extra flour mixture, then let it alone for ten to fifteen minutes.

2. In a good pan over medium heat, liquefy 1 tablespoon of coconut oil. For one minute, sauté the garlic, ginger powder, and red pepper flakes.

3. Add the coconut aminos, honey, and broth and mix to thoroughly blend. Cook for three minutes on high heat while stirring periodically. Turn off the heat and let the pot alone.

4. Heat the remaining coconut oil in a big skillet over medium heat, then stir-fry the beef for two to three minutes. Stir-fry for a minute in the skillet's remaining oil.

5. After 3 minutes of cooking, stir in the honey sauce. After adding the scallion, cook for another minute. Serve hot.

**Nutritional Info:** Calories 333; Fat 15.2g; Carbs 3.1g; Protein 43.6g; Fiber 0.6g

## Garlicky Broiled Lamb Shoulder

Time to prepare: 10 minutes + marinating time
Time to cook: 10 minutes
Servings: 6

Ingredients

- 2 lb. grass-fed lamb shoulder, trimmed
- ¼ cup fresh lemongrass stalk, minced
- ¼ cup fresh orange juice
- ¼ cup coconut aminos
- 2 tablespoon fresh ginger, minced
- 2 tablespoon garlic, minced
- Ground black pepper to taste

**Directions:**

1. Combine all the ingredients in a bowl, excluding the lamb shoulder.

2. Arrange the lamb shoulder in your baking dish and generously brush the lamb with half of the marinade mixture. Keep the leftover mixture aside. overnight marinating in the refrigerator.

3. Set the broiler oven's rack 5 inches away from the heating element and preheat it. Shake off the excess marinade before removing the lamb shoulder from the refrigerator.

4. Broil each side for 4-5 minutes. Serve with the marinade you set aside.

**Nutritional Info:** Calories 341; Fat 17.6g; Carbs 5.3g; Protein 37.6g; Fiber 0.3 g

## Spiced Lamb Chops

Time to prepare: 10 minutes
Time to cook: 6 minutes
Servings: 4

**Ingredients:**

- 8 grass-fed medium lamb chops, trimmed
- 4 garlic cloves, peeled
- 1 tablespoon coconut oil
- 1 teaspoon black mustard seeds, crushed finely
- 2 teaspoon ground cumin

- 1 teaspoon ground ginger
- 1 teaspoon ground coriander
- ½ teaspoon ground cinnamon
- Salt & ground black pepper to taste

**Directions:**

1. Spread some salt on a cutting board and add the garlic cloves. Crush the garlic with a knife until you have a paste.
2. Combine spices and garlic paste in a bowl. With a sharp knife, score the chops three to four times on each side. Apply the garlic mixture liberally to the chops.
3. Cook the chops for 5 minutes on each side after melting the coconut oil in a skillet. Serve hot.

**Nutritional Info:** Calories 494; Fat 15.7g; Carbs 2.3g; Protein 84.8g; Fiber 0.5g

## Pork Tenderloin with Dijon-Cider Glaze

Time to prepare: 10 minutes
Time to cook: 25 minutes
Servings: 4

**Ingredients:**

- 1 (1½ lb.) pork tenderloin
- ¼ cup apple cider vinegar
- ¼ cup coconut sugar
- 3 tablespoon Dijon mustard
- 2 teaspoon garlic powder
- Dash of salt

**Directions:**

1. Stir the salt, vinegar, mustard, garlic powder, and coconut sugar in a small bowl until the sugar dissolves. Brush the pork loin with this mixture.
2. Place the meat on your grill pan and preheat it to medium-high. 2 minutes per side for searing
3. Spoon the pork with half of the vinegar mixture, then turn the heat down to medium. Cook for 10 minutes with the cover on.
4. Drizzle the meat with the remaining vinegar mixture. The pork should be cooked for 5 minutes, or until the center registers 145°F.
5. Place the platter with the meat on it. Simmer the vinegar mixture that is still in the pan. For a reduction and thickening, cook for 5 minutes. Serve the pork with the glaze poured over it.

**Nutritional Info:** Calories: 268; Fat: 6g; Carbs: 16g; Protein: 36g; Fiber: 0g

## Garlicky Lamb Stew

Time to prepare: 10 minutes
Time to cook: 15 minutes
Servings: 4

**Ingredients:**

- 1 lb. ground lamb
- 1 (28 oz) can of chopped tomatoes, drained (no seeds)
- 5 garlic cloves, minced
- 1 onion, chopped
- 1 tablespoon extra-virgin olive oil
- 1 teaspoon dried oregano
- ½ teaspoon sea salt
- ¼ teaspoon freshly ground black pepper

**Directions:**

1. Cook the lamb for approximately 5 minutes over medium-high heat in your big nonstick pan, crumbling the meat with a wooden spoon as it cooks.
2. Remove the lamb from the dish after draining the fat. Put the skillet back on the burner, add the oil, and heat it until it shimmers.
3. Include the onion, oregano, pepper, and salt. To soften the onions, cook and stir for 5 minutes.
4. Add the tomatoes and add the lamb back to the skillet. Cook for 3 minutes, stirring once or twice, or until well heated.
5. Stir continuously for 30 seconds after adding the garlic. Serve!

**Nutritional Info:** Calories: 295; Fat: 12g; Protein: 34g; Carbs: 12g; Fiber: 3g

## Pork with Pears and Ginger

Time to prepare: 10 minutes
Time to cook: 35 minutes
Servings: 4

**Ingredients:**
- 2 lb. pork roast, sliced
- 2 pears, peeled, cored & cut into wedges
- 2 green onions, chopped
- 2 tablespoon avocado oil
- ½ tablespoon coconut aminos
- 1 tablespoon ginger, minced
- ¼ cup vegetable stock
- 1 tablespoon chives, chopped

**Directions:**
1. Heat the oil in a pan over medium heat. Cook the meat for two minutes on each side after adding the onions.
2. Add the remaining ingredients, gently toss, and bake for 30 minutes at 390°F. Serve the mixture by dividing it among plates.

**Nutritional Info:** Calories 220; Fat 13.3g; Carbs 16.5g; Protein 8g; Fiber 2g

## Lamb Meatballs

Time to prepare: 15 minutes
Time to cook: 20 minutes
Servings: 4

**Ingredients:**
- 1½ lb. ground lamb
- 2 tablespoon dried rosemary leaves
- 1 tablespoon dried oregano
- 1 teaspoon onion powder
- 1 teaspoon garlic powder
- ½ teaspoon sea salt
- ¼ teaspoon freshly ground black pepper

**Directions:**
1. Turn on the oven to 400°F.
2. In a large bowl, combine the lamb, rosemary, oregano, onion powder, garlic powder, salt, and pepper.
3. Form the mixture into 20 (3/4-inch) balls, and then place them on a baking sheet with a rim. After 20 minutes of baking, serve.

**Nutritional Info:** Calories: 445; Fat: 23g; Carbs: 10g; Protein: 48g; Fibers: 1g

## Garlicky Bolognese Pork Zoodles

Time to prepare: 10 minutes
Time to cook: 25 minutes
Servings: 3

**Ingredients:**
- ¾ lb. ground pork
- 3 teaspoon olive oil
- 2 cloves garlic, pressed
- 2 medium-sized tomatoes, peeled, seeded & puréed
- 2 zucchinis, peeled, seeded & spiralized

**Directions:**
1. In a saucepan set over medium-high heat, warm the olive oil. Pork should not be pink after 3 to 4 minutes of searing after the pan is heated.
2. Add the garlic and stir. Cook for an additional 30 seconds, or until fragrant. Add the puréed tomatoes after boiling them. Within 20 minutes, simmer over medium-low heat.
3. Stir in the zoodles, then cook for 112 minutes, or until they are just al dente. Serve warm.

**Nutritional Info:** Calories: 358; Fat: 28.6g; Carbs: 4.0g; Protein: 20.2g; Fiber: 1.2g

## Herbed Ribeye Steak

Time to prepare: 10 minutes
Time to cook: 10 minutes
Servings: 4

**Ingredients:**

- 4 small or 2 large (halved) 1½-inch-thick rib-eye steaks, salted 2 to 24 hours before cooking
- 7 tablespoon olive oil, divided
- 4 teaspoon fresh chopped basil leaves
- 1 teaspoon fresh chopped thyme leaves
- ½ teaspoon garlic powder
- Salt & ground black pepper to taste

**Directions:**

1. Turn on the low broiler.
2. In a large oven-safe skillet, heat 3 tablespoons of oil over medium-high heat.
3. Pat the steaks dry and season with salt and pepper as you wait.
4. To get a dark sear, cook the steaks in the pan for 1 to 2 minutes. To get a dark sear on the second side of your steaks, flip them over and sear for one to two minutes.
5. To cook a medium-rare steak, place the pan in a hot oven and broil for two to three minutes before turning.
6. Remove and set aside for 5 minutes to allow the fluids to disperse.
7. In a separate dish, combine the remaining 4 tablespoon of oil, basil, thyme, and garlic powder.
8. Spoon equal portions of the mixture over the steak before serving.

**Nutritional Info:** Calories: 593; Fat: 44g; Carbs: 4g; Protein: 46g; Fiber: 1g

## Herb-Crusted Racks of Lamb

Time to prepare: 10 minutes
Time to cook: 25 minutes
Servings: 4

**Ingredients:**

- 2 racks of lamb (8 ribs each), at room temperature

For the herb seasoning:

- 1 medium onion, finely chopped
- ¼ cup gluten-free fine bread crumbs
- 2 teaspoon minced fresh oregano
- 1 tablespoon chopped fresh dill
- 1 teaspoon salt
- 1/8 teaspoon freshly ground black pepper

**Directions:**

1. Turn the oven on to 425 °F.
2. In a bowl, combine all the seasoning ingredients. The lamb should be seasoned.
3. Arrange the lamb in a roasting pan on a broiler rack. In less than 25 minutes, roast for medium rare.

**Nutritional Info:** Calories: 579; Fat: 44g; Carbs: 13g; Protein: 33g; Fiber: 1g

## Pan Seared Salmon

Time to prepare: 10 minutes
Time to cook: 9 minutes
Servings: 4
**Ingredients:**
- 4 (4-oz.) salmon fillets
- 2 tablespoon olive oil
- Salt & ground black pepper to taste

**Directions:**
1. Evenly season the salmon fillets with salt and pepper.
2. Heat the oil over medium heat in a nonstick pan. Salmon fillets should be cooked skin side down for about 3–5 minutes without stirring.
3. After about 3–4 minutes of cooking, flip the salmon fillets. Serve warm.

**Nutritional Info:** Calories: 261; Fat: 19g; Carbs: 0g; Protein: 22.1g; Fiber: 0g

## Parsley Salmon

Time to prepare: 10 minutes
Time to cook: 20 minutes
Servings: 6
**Ingredients:**
- 6 (4-oz.) salmon fillets
- 3 tablespoon fresh parsley, minced
- 2 tablespoon olive oil
- Salt & ground black pepper to taste

**Directions:**
1. Preheat the oven to 400°F and butter a large baking pan.
2. Combine all the ingredients in a dish and stir well. Put your baking dish with the salmon fillets in a single layer.
3. Bake to the desired doneness in 15 to 20 minutes. Serve.

**Nutritional Info:** Calories: 191; Fat: 11.7g; Carbs: 0.1g; Protein: 22.1g; Fiber: 0.1g

## Honey Parsley Salmon

Time to prepare: 10 minutes
Time to cook: 8 minutes
Servings: 4
**Ingredients:**
- 4 (4-oz.) skinless salmon fillets
- 2 tablespoon olive oil
- 2 tablespoon fresh parsley, chopped
- 1 tablespoon organic honey
- 1 tablespoon fresh lemon juice

**Directions:**
1. Combine the honey and lemon juice in your bowl. Place aside.
2. Cook the salmon fillets in the olive oil for approximately 3 to 4 minutes on each side in a large nonstick sauté pan. Add the honey mixture, and then serve right away.

**Nutritional Info:** Calories: 278; Fat: 19.1g; Carbs: 4.5g; Protein: 22.2g; Fiber: 0.1g

## Salmon Parcel

Time to prepare: 10 minutes
Time to cook: 20 minutes
Servings: 6
**Ingredients:**
- 6 (3-oz.) salmon fillets
- 2 bell peppers, seeded & cubed (if tolerated)
- 4 tomatoes, peeled, seeded & cubed
- ½ cup fresh parsley, chopped
- 2 tablespoon olive oil
- 2 tablespoon fresh lemon juice
- Salt & ground black pepper to taste

**Directions:**
1. Set your oven's temperature to 400°F and lay six pieces of foil out on a flat surface.
2. Arrange 1 salmon fillet per foil paper;

season with salt and pepper.

3. Combine the bell peppers and tomatoes in your bowl.

4. Evenly distribute the vegetable mixture over each fillet, then garnish with capers and parsley. Add oil and lemon juice to the dish.

5. To seal the salmon mixture, fold the foil over itself. Place the foil packets in a single layer on a sizable baking sheet. For 20 minutes, bake. Serve warm.

**Nutritional Info:** Calories: 178; Fat: 10.2g; Carbs: 5.5g; Protein: 17.8g; Fiber: 1.8g

## Salmon In Tomato Sauce

Time to prepare: 10 minutes
Time to cook: 8 minutes
Servings: 6
**Ingredients:**
- 1½ lb. skinless salmon fillets, cubed into 2-inch size
- 3 cups tomatoes, peeled, seeded & chopped
- 1¼ cup homemade chicken broth
- 2 tablespoon fresh parsley, chopped
- 1 tablespoon olive oil
- Salt to taste

**Directions:**
1. In your large pan, heat the oil over medium heat. Once the oil is hot, add the tomatoes and cook, crushing them with the back of a spoon, for about 2–3 minutes.

2. After adding the broth, gently boil. Salmon pieces are added and cooked for about 4–5 minutes. Serve hot after adding the salt and basil leaves.

**Nutritional Info:** Calories: 245; Fat: 14.8g; Carbs: 3.8g; Protein: 24g; Fiber: 1.1g

## Salmon & Spinach Soup

Time to prepare: 10 minutes
Time to cook: 30 minutes
Servings: 8
**Ingredients:**
- 1½ lb. salmon fillets, cubed
- 8 cups homemade chicken broth
- 2 cups carrots, peeled & chopped
- 8 cups fresh baby spinach
- 1 cup fresh cilantro, chopped
- Salt to taste

**Directions:**
1. Place a large soup pot over high heat and add the carrots and broth. Simmer for about 15 minutes after adjusting the heat to medium-low.

2. Add the salmon cubes, spinach, cilantro, and salt, and simmer for 10 to 15 minutes with the lid on. Serve warm.

**Nutritional Info:** Calories: 170; Fat: 6.8g; Carbs: 4.8g; Protein: 22.5g; Fiber: 1.3g

## Herbed Swordfish

Time to prepare: 10 minutes
Time to cook: 8 minutes
Servings: 2
**Ingredients:**
- 2 (6-oz.) swordfish steaks
- 2 tablespoon orange zest, grated
- 1 tablespoon fresh thyme, chopped
- 1 tablespoon fresh parsley, chopped
- 1 teaspoon olive oil

**Directions:**
1. Set your oven's broiler to high.

2. Combine oil, herbs, and orange zest in a bowl. Generously rub the herb mixture into the fish steaks.

3. Place the fish steaks on a broiler pan and cook for 3 to 4 minutes on each side. Serve warm.

**Nutritional Info:** Calories: 29; Fat: 11.2g; Carbs: 2.5g; Protein: 43.5g; Fiber: 1.2g

## Simple Tilapia Soup

Time to prepare: 10 minutes
Time to cook: 7 minutes
Servings: 5

**Ingredients:**

- 5 (5-oz.) tilapia fillets
- 2 tablespoon olive oil
- 4 cups homemade chicken broth
- Salt & ground black pepper to taste

**Directions:**

1. Heat oil in a large sauté pan over medium heat before adding the tilapia fillets and cooking for about 3 minutes total. Cook for about 1–2 minutes after flipping.
2. Include the broth and cook for an additional 2 to 3 minutes. Serve hot after adding salt and pepper to taste.

**Nutritional Info:** Calories: 167; Fat: 7g; Carbs: 0.1g; Protein: 26.6g; Fiber: 0g

## Haddock In Tomato Sauce

Time to prepare: 10 minutes
Time to cook: 20 minutes
Servings: 3

**Ingredients:**

- 3 (4-oz.) haddock fillets
- 2½ cups tomatoes, peeled, seeded & chopped
- 3 tablespoon fresh cilantro, chopped
- 1 tablespoon olive oil
- 1 tablespoon balsamic vinegar
- Salt & ground black pepper to taste

**Directions:**

1. Set the oven to 325°F.
2. In a medium, oven-safe non-stick sauté pan, heat oil over medium heat. While stirring frequently, saute the tomatoes for approximately 2 minutes.
3. Add the vinegar and cilantro, and simmer for two to three minutes. Stir in

the haddock fillets, salt, and pepper before adding them to the sauce.
4. Bake the sauté pan for 12 to 15 minutes in the oven. Serve warm.

**Nutritional Info:** Calories: 195; Fat: 6g; Carbs: 5.9g; Protein: 28.8g; Fiber: 1.7g

## Tomato Cod Potato Soup

Time to prepare: 10 minutes
Time to cook: 20-25 minutes
Servings: 5

**Ingredients:**

- 1¼ lb. cod, cut into bite-sized chunks
- 3 cups homemade chicken broth
- 2 cups potatoes, peeled & chopped
- 2 cups tomatoes, peeled, seeded & chopped
- 2 cups water
- 2 tablespoon fresh parsley, chopped
- Salt & ground black pepper to taste

**Directions:**

1. Place a large soup pot over medium-high heat and bring the potatoes, tomatoes, broth, and water to a boil.
2. Adjust the heat to low and simmer for 10 to 15 minutes.
3. Add the cod and cook for 4-5 minutes, stirring gently every so often. Serve immediately after adding the parsley, salt, and black pepper.

**Nutritional Info:** Calories: 181; Fat: 2g; Carbs: 15.9g; Protein: 24.9g; Fiber: 2g

## Lemony Trout

Time to prepare: 10 minutes
Time to cook: 25 minutes
Servings: 8

**Ingredients:**

- 2 (1½-lb.) trout, gutted & cleaned
- 1 lemon, sliced
- 2 tablespoon fresh dill, minced
- 2 tablespoon olive oil

- 2 tablespoon fresh lemon juice
- Salt & ground black pepper to taste

**Directions:**

1. Set a wire rack on a baking sheet that has been lined with foil while preheating your oven to 475°F.
2. Liberally season the trout with black pepper and salt, both inside and out. Each fish's cavity should be filled with lemon and dill.
3. Spread the melted butter and lemon juice over the trout before placing it on the prepared baking sheet.
4. After 25 minutes of baking, take the baking sheet out and put the trout on a serving platter. Serve warm.

**Nutritional Info:** Calories: 300; Fat: 16.9g; Carbs: 0.7g; Protein: 36.7g; Fiber: 0.2g

## Shrimp With Bell Peppers

Time to prepare: 10 minutes
Time to cook: 10 minutes
Servings: 5

**Ingredients:**

- 1 lb. medium shrimp, peeled & deveined
- 3 cups bell peppers, seeded & julienned
- ¼ cup homemade chicken broth
- 2 tablespoon olive oil
- Salt & ground black pepper to taste

**Directions:**

1. Heat the olive oil in a sizable nonstick sauté pan over medium heat, then cook the bell peppers for about 3 to 4 minutes.
2. Stir-fry the shrimp for 3–4 minutes while adding salt and black pepper. Add broth and cook for a few minutes after stirring. Serve warm.

**Nutritional Info:** Calories: 147; Fat: 6.8g; Carbs: 2.6g; Protein: 20.2g; Fiber: 0.9g

## Shrimp With Asparagus

Time to prepare: 10 minutes
Time to cook: 11 minutes
Servings: 6

**Ingredients:**

- 1 lb. shrimp, peeled and deveined
- 1 lb. asparagus tips
- 3 tablespoon olive oil, divided
- 1 tablespoon dried parsley
- Salt & ground black pepper to taste

**Directions:**

1. In a sizable sauté pan with 1 tablespoon oil heated to medium-high, stir-fry the asparagus for 4–5 minutes. The asparagus should be placed on a plate.
2. In the same sauté pan with the remaining oil, stir-fry the shrimp for 2 minutes. For about a minute, add parsley, salt, and black pepper.
3. Add the cooked asparagus and cook for an additional two to three minutes. Serve warm.

**Nutritional Info:** Calories: 168; Fat: 8.3g; Carbs: 3.6g; Protein: 19.1g; Fiber: 1.2g

## Shrimp With Zucchini

Time to prepare: 10 minutes
Time to cook: 10 minutes
Servings: 6

**Ingredients:**

- 1¼ lb. shrimp, peeled & deveined
- 3 zucchinis, peeled, seeded & chopped
- ¼ cup tomatoes, peeled, seeded & chopped
- 1/3 cup homemade chicken broth
- 2 tablespoon olive oil
- Salt & ground black pepper to taste

**Directions:**

1. In a cast-iron skillet, heat the olive oil over medium heat. Cook the zucchini for two to three minutes.
2. Cook the shrimp for about 2 minutes after adding salt and black pepper. Cook

for three to five minutes after adding the broth and tomatoes. Serve warm.
**Nutritional Info:** Calories: 171; Fat: 6.6g; Carbs: 5.1g; Protein: 23.1g; Fiber: 1.2g

## Shrimp Zucchini Soup

Time to prepare: 10 minutes
Time to cook: 23 minutes
Servings: 4
**Ingredients:**
- 1 lb. shrimp, peeled and deveined
- 2 cups zucchini, peeled, seeded & sliced
- 3½ cups homemade chicken broth
- 2 tablespoon olive oil
- 2 tablespoon fresh parsley, minced
- Salt & ground black pepper to taste

**Directions:**
1. In your skillet, heat the oil over medium heat. Cook the zucchini, stirring frequently, for about 2–3 minutes.
2. Add the broth, then simmer for 10 to 15 minutes.
3. Include the shrimp, season with salt and black pepper, and simmer for 4-5 minutes. Add the parsley and serve immediately.

**Nutritional Info:** Calories: 235; Fat: 10.2g; Carbs: 4.5g; Protein: 30.8g; Fiber: 0.7g

## Shrimp Stew

Time to prepare: 10 minutes
Time to cook: 9 minutes
Servings: 6
**Ingredients:**
- 1½ lb. raw shrimp, peeled & deveined
- 3 cups tomatoes, peeled, seeded & chopped
- 1 cup homemade chicken broth
- 2 tablespoon olive oil
- 2 tablespoon fresh lime juice

- 2 tablespoon fresh cilantro, chopped
- Salt & ground black pepper to taste

**Directions:**
1. Add the shrimp and tomatoes to the pan with the oil already heated over medium heat, and cook for 3–4 minutes.
2. Add the broth and stir; cook for 4-5 minutes. Remove from the heat after adding the lime juice, salt, and black pepper. Serve hot with cilantro as a garnish.

**Nutritional Info:** Calories: 200; Fat: 7g; Carbs: 5.9g; Protein: 27.5g; Fiber: 1.2g

## Creamy Prawns

Time to prepare: 10 minutes
Time to cook: 7 minutes
Servings: 4
**Ingredients:**
- 1 lb. prawns, peeled & deveined
- ¾ cup unsweetened coconut milk
- 2 tablespoon olive oil
- 2 tablespoon fresh basil, chopped
- Salt & ground black pepper to taste

**Directions:**
1. Heat the oil in a large sauté pan over medium heat before cooking the prawns for 1-2 minutes. Stir in the coconut milk slowly.
2. Let simmer for four to five minutes. Basil, salt, and black pepper should also be added at this point. Serve warm.

**Nutritional Info:** Calories: 263; Fat: 15.1g; Carbs: 2.9g; Protein: 26.4g; Fiber: 0g

## Scallops With Zucchini

Time to prepare: 10 minutes
Time to cook: 10 minutes
Servings: 3
**Ingredients:**
- ¾ lb. scallops

- 2 cups zucchini, peeled, seeded & chopped
- 2 tablespoon olive oil
- 1 teaspoon fresh lemon juice
- Salt to taste

**Directions:**

1. In a large sauté pan, heat the oil over medium heat. Cook the zucchini, stirring occasionally, for about 3 to 5 minutes.
2. Add the scallops and cook for 3 to 4 minutes, flipping halfway through.
3. After adding the lemon juice, turn off the heat. Serve warm.

**Nutritional Info:** Calories: 192; Fat: 10.3g; Carbs: 5.2g; Protein: 20g; Fiber: 0.8g

## Cilantro Lemon Shrimp

Time to prepare: 20 minutes + marinating time
Time to cook: 6 minutes
Servings: 4

**Ingredients:**

- 1 ½ lb. large shrimp, deveined & shells removed
- 4 garlic cloves
- 1 cup fresh cilantro leaves
- ½ cup lemon juice
- ½ teaspoon ground coriander
- 3 tablespoon extra-virgin olive oil
- 1 teaspoon salt

**Directions:**

1. Blend the salt, olive oil, garlic, cilantro, and coriander in a food processor until smooth.
2. Pour the cilantro marinade over the shrimp and let it sit for 15 minutes in a bowl or plastic zip-top bag.
3. Heat a skillet to a high temperature. In the skillet, add the shrimp and marinade. For three minutes on each side, cook the shrimp. Serve hot.

**Nutritional Info:** Calories: 225; Fat: 12g; Carbs: 5g; Protein: 28g; Fiber: 0.5g

## Seafood Risotto

Time to prepare: 15 minutes
Time to cook: 30 minutes
Servings: 4

**Ingredients:**

- 8 oz shrimp, peeled & deveined
- 8 oz scallops
- 3 garlic cloves, minced
- 1 large onion, chopped
- 6 cups vegetable broth
- 1 ½ cups arborio rice
- 3 tablespoon extra-virgin olive oil
- ½ teaspoon saffron threads
- 1 ½ teaspoon salt

**Directions:**

1. In a large saucepan over medium heat, simmer the broth.
2. Cook the onion, garlic, saffron, and olive oil in a large skillet for 3 minutes over medium heat.
3. Pour 1 cup of broth into the pan along with the rice and salt. Stir thoroughly, then simmer until the majority of the liquid has been absorbed.
4. Carry out the steps again using broth, adding 12 cups at a time and cooking until all but 12 cups of the broth are absorbed.
5. After stirring the last 1/2 cup of broth, add the shrimp and scallops. Cook for 10 minutes with a cover on. Serve hot.

**Nutritional Info:** Calories: 460; Fat: 12g; Carbs: 64g; Protein: 24g; Fiber: 0.6g

## Fast Seafood Paella

Time to prepare: 15 minutes
Time to cook: 20 minutes
Servings: 4

**Ingredients:**

- 8 oz lobster meat or canned crab
- 6 jumbo shrimp, unpeeled
- 1 lb. calamari rings

- 2 tomatoes, peeled, seeded & chopped
- 2 carrots, peeled & finely diced
- 1 large onion, finely chopped
- 3 cups chicken stock, + more if needed
- 1 ½ cups medium-grain arborio rice
- 1 cup dry white wine
- ½ cup frozen peas
- ¼ cup + 1 tablespoon extra-virgin olive oil
- 1 ½ tablespoon garlic powder
- 1 lemon, halved
- Salt, to taste

**Directions:**

1. In a sizable skillet or sauté pan, heat the oil over medium heat. After 3 minutes of cooking the onion until fragrant, add the tomatoes and garlic powder.

2. Cook the tomatoes for 5 to 10 minutes, or until they have reduced by half. Rice, carrots, salt, lobster, and peas are all added and thoroughly mixed.

3. Heat the chicken stock to almost boiling in a pot or microwave-safe bowl before adding it to the rice mixture. After letting it boil, add the wine.

4. Even out the rice in the pan's bottom. For 10 minutes, cook covered over low heat while stirring occasionally to prevent burning.

5. Place the shrimp on top of the rice, cover it, and cook for an additional 5 minutes. Add the calamari rings, take them out, and keep tossing the ingredients.

6. Add some freshly squeezed lemon juice and serve.

**Nutritional Info:** Calories: 632; Fat: 20g; Carbs: 71g; Protein: 34g; Fiber: 0.6g

### Crispy Fried Sardines

Time to prepare: 5 minutes
Time to cook: 6 minutes
Servings: 4

**Ingredients:**

- 1 ½ lb. whole fresh sardines, scales removed
- 2 cups refined flour
- 1 teaspoon salt
- 1 teaspoon freshly ground black pepper
- Avocado oil, as needed

**Directions:**

1. Heat a deep skillet over medium heat.Enough oil should be added before seasoning the fish with salt and pepper.

2. Coat the fish thoroughly with flour before dredging. Cook the fish for 3 minutes on each side, or until it starts to brown. Serve hot.

**Nutritional Info:** Calories: 794; Fat: 47g; Carbs: 44g; Protein: 48g; Fiber: 3.2g

### Shrimp with Garlic and Mushrooms

Time to prepare: 15 minutes
Time to cook: 15 minutes
Servings: 4

**Ingredients:**

- 1 lb. fresh shrimp, peeled & deveined
- 1 teaspoon salt
- 1 cup extra-virgin olive oil
- 8 large garlic cloves, thinly sliced
- 4 oz sliced mushrooms
- ¼ cup chopped fresh flat-leaf Italian parsley

**Directions:**

1. Add salt to your bowl before adding the shrimp. In a large, thick-rimmed skillet over medium heat, warm the olive oil.

2. After adding it, cook the garlic for 3 to 4 minutes, or until it is very fragrant.

3. Include the mushrooms and cook for 5 minutes, or until they are soft. In 3 to 4 minutes, add the shrimp and simmer until it starts to turn pink.

4. Take out and add the parsley. Serve!

**Nutritional Info:** Calories: 620; Fat: 56g; Carbs: 4g; Protein: 24g; Fiber: 1g

## Mussels in Curried Coconut Milk

Time to prepare: 10 minutes
Time to cook: 15 minutes
Servings: 4

**Ingredients:**
- 1½ lb. fresh mussels, scrubbed & debearded
- ½ sweet onion, finely chopped
- 1 cup coconut milk
- 2 tablespoon olive oil
- 2 tablespoon finely chopped cilantro
- 1 tablespoon minced garlic
- 1 tablespoon curry powder
- 2 teaspoon grated fresh ginger

**Directions:**
1. In a large skillet over medium-high heat, add the olive oil and cook the onion, garlic, and ginger for about 3 minutes, or until they are soft.
2. Include the curry powder and blend by tossing. Add the coconut milk and stir before bringing it to a boil.
3. Add the mussels, cover, and steam for 8 minutes or until the shells are open. Turn off the heat and take out any shells that haven't been cracked. Add the cilantro, and then serve.

**Nutritional Info:** Calories: 263; Fat: 23g; Carbs: 9g; Protein: 9g; Fiber: 2g

## Classic Blackened Scallops

Time to prepare: 10 minutes
Time to cook: 3 minutes
Servings: 4

**Ingredients:**
- 1 lb. sea scallops, cleaned
- 2 tablespoon olive oil
- 2 teaspoon onion powder
- 1 teaspoon garlic powder
- 1 teaspoon sea salt
- 1 teaspoon dried thyme
- ½ teaspoon freshly ground black pepper

**Directions:**
1. Combine the salt, pepper, thyme, onion powder, and garlic powder in a small bowl.
2. After drying the scallops with a paper towel, dredge both the top and bottom of the scallops in the spice mixture.
3. Heat the olive oil in a large skillet over medium-high heat. Making sure they don't touch, add the scallops to the skillet.
4. For about 3 minutes, sear both sides while turning once.

**Nutritional Info:** Calories: 178; Fat: 8g; Carbs: 6g; Protein: 20g; Fiber: 2g

## Soused Herring

Time to prepare: 10 minutes
Time to cook: 30 minutes
Servings: 4

**Ingredients:**
- 4 whole herring fillets, scaled, filleted, & trimmed
- 2 cups water
- ½ sweet onion, thinly sliced
- ½ cup white vinegar
- 2 thyme sprigs
- 1 tablespoon granulated stevia
- 1 teaspoon sea salt
- ¼ teaspoon black peppercorns

**Directions:**
1. Set the oven's temperature to 350°F. In a baking dish measuring 9 by 13 inches, put the herring fillets.
2. Include the peppercorns, sugar, salt, onion, white vinegar, and water. Bake the fish for 25 to 30 minutes, until it is tender, in a covered baking dish. Prior to serving, cool

**Nutritional Info:** Calories: 277; Fat: 15g; Carbs: 5g; Protein: 29g; Fiber: 0g

## Steamed Garlic-Dill Halibut

Time to prepare: 5 Minutes
Time to cook: 25 Minutes
Servings: 4

**Ingredients:**
- 1 lb. halibut fillet
- 1 lemon, freshly squeezed
- 1 tablespoon dill weed, chopped
- 1 teaspoon garlic powder
- Salt & pepper to taste
- Water, as needed

**Directions:**

1. Add enough water to your big pot and bring it up to medium. In the saucepan, set your trivet.

2. Place all the ingredients in your baking dish and stir well. The dish is covered with foil. Place your trivet inside the pot and the dish on top of it.

3. For 15 minutes, steam fish in a covered saucepan. Before removing it from the pot, give it 10 minutes to rest. Enjoy after serving.

**Nutritional Info:** Calories 270; Fat 6.5g; Carbs 3.9g; Protein 47.8g; Fiber 2.1g

## Zucchini Pasta with Shrimp

Time to prepare: 15 minutes
Time to cook: 7 minutes
Servings: 4

**Ingredients:**
- 1 lb. shrimp, peeled and deveined
- 4 large zucchinis, peeled, seeded & spiralized
- 2 tablespoon coconut oil
- 1 tablespoon extra-virgin olive oil
- 3 garlic cloves, minced
- 4 to 6 fresh basil leaves, chopped
- Salt & pepper to taste

**Directions:**

1. In a large skillet, heat the coconut and olive oils over medium heat. Sauté for one minute after adding the garlic.

2. Include the shrimp and cook for two to three minutes. Cook the zucchini for two to three minutes, occasionally tossing.

3. Add salt and black pepper, then turn the heat off. Basil leaves should be used as a garnish when serving.

**Nutritional Info:** Calories: 59; Fat: 1g; Carbs: 14g; Protein: 1g; Fiber: 1g

## Shrimp Scampi

Time to prepare: 10 minutes
Time to cook: 15 minutes
Servings: 2

**Ingredients:**
- 1 lb. shrimp, peeled and tails removed
- 3 minced garlic cloves
- 1 lemon zest
- ½ chopped red bell pepper
- ½ finely chopped onion
- 1 lemon juice
- 2 tablespoon extra-virgin olive oil
- ¼ teaspoon sea salt
- A pinch of freshly ground black pepper

**Directions:**

1. In a sizable nonstick pan, heat the olive oil over medium-high heat until

2. Include the onion and red bell pepper. Cook until tender, stirring frequently, for about 6 minutes.

3. Cook the shrimp for about 5 minutes, or until they turn yellow. Include the garlic. Stirring constantly, cook for 30 seconds.

4. Add the lemon juice, pepper, salt, and zest. 3 minutes of cooking at low heat Serve!

**Nutritional Info:** Calories: 345; Fat: 16g; Carbs: 10g; Protein: 40g; Fiber: 1g

## Shrimp with Cinnamon Sauce

Time to prepare: 5 minutes
Time to cook: 10 minutes
Servings: 2

**Ingredients:**

- 1 lb. shrimp, peeled
- ½ cup no-salt-added chicken broth
- 1 tablespoon extra-virgin olive oil
- 1 tablespoon Dijon Mustard
- ½ teaspoon ground cinnamon
- ½ teaspoon onion powder
- ½ teaspoon ground black pepper
- ¼ teaspoon sea salt

**Directions:**

1. In a large nonstick skillet over medium-high heat, warm the olive oil until it shimmers.

2. Add the shrimp. Cook for 4 minutes, stirring often, or until opaque.

3. In a shallow cup, combine the chicken broth, mustard, onion powder, salt, cinnamon, and pepper. Pour this into the skillet and cook for another three minutes, stirring frequently.

**Nutritional Info:** Calories: 270; Fat: 11g; Carbs: 4g; Protein: 39g; Fiber: 1g

## Steamed Lemon Pepper Salmon

Time to prepare: 10 minutes
Time to cook: 20 minutes
Servings: 4

**Ingredients:**

- 4 salmon fillets
- 2 tablespoon olive oil
- 2 tablespoon soy sauce
- 1 teaspoon lemon juice
- Salt & pepper to taste

**Directions:**

1. Set a trivet or steamer basket inside your pot, then fill it with water to a height of 1 inch. Make it boil.

2. To fit in the pot, arrange the salmon fillets in your baking dish. Pour the remaining ingredients on top. Mix thoroughly, then tightly wrap the dish in foil.

3. Place the steam rack on top of your baking dish. For 15 minutes, close the lid and steam the fish. After the fish has cooled for five minutes, turn off the heat. Enjoy after serving.

**Nutritional Info:** Calories 239; Fat 16.7g; Carbs 0.9g; Protein 20.2g; Fiber 0.3g

## Apple and Mushroom Soup

Time to prepare: 5 minutes
Time to cook: 5 minutes
Servings: 2
**Ingredients:**
- ½ green apple, peeled, cored, & grated
- 3 ½ oz silken tofu, crumbled
- 3 oz pre-cooked refined rice noodles
- 2 mushrooms, sliced
- 1 1/2 cup water
- ¼ cup green chives, chopped
- 1 slice roasted seaweed, crushed

**Directions:**
1. In a skillet, combine all the ingredients (seaweed flakes not included) and heat for 1-2 minutes while stirring.
2. Serve after adding the seaweed flakes!

**Nutritional Info:** Calories: 366; Fat: 19g; Carbs: 41.1g; Proteins: 11g; Fibers: 3g

## Cantaloupe Gazpacho

Time to prepare: 10 minutes + chilling time
Time to cook: 0 minutes
Servings: 4
**Ingredients:**
- 2 cantaloupes, seeded, peeled, & diced
- 1 English cucumber, peeled, seeded & diced
- 2 shallots, finely chopped
- 1 tablespoon apple cider vinegar

**Directions:**
1. Blend the cantaloupes, cucumber, vinegar, and shallots in a food processor until smooth.
2. Transfer the soup to your container and chill for approximately one hour in the fridge. Serve.

**Nutritional Info:** Calories: 155; Fat: 1g; Carbs: 37g; Protein: 4g; Fiber: 4g

## Shrimp Ginger Soup

Time to prepare: 10 minutes
Time to cook: 20 minutes
Servings: 4
**Ingredients:**
- 1 lb. shrimp, peeled, deveined, & chopped into ¼-inch pieces
- 3 cups low-sodium vegetable stock
- 2 cups shredded kale
- 1 cup full-fat coconut milk
- 1 tablespoon olive oil
- 2 teaspoon minced garlic
- 2 teaspoon grated fresh ginger
- Sea salt & ground black pepper to taste

**Directions:**
1. Heat the olive oil in a large saucepan over medium heat. For approximately 2 minutes, sauté the ginger and garlic until they are tender.
2. Include the coconut milk and vegetable stock. Shrimp and greens are added after allowing it to boil.
3. Lower the heat to low and simmer the soup for five minutes, or until the shrimp is nearly done. Serve right after adding salt and pepper to taste.

**Nutritional Info:** Calories: 309; Fat: 19g; Carbs: 9g; Protein: 26g; Fiber: 2g

## Miso Whitefish Soup with Chard

Time to prepare: 10 minutes
Time to cook: 15 minutes
Servings: 4
**Ingredients:**
- 1 lb. whitefish, thinly sliced
- 6 cups low-sodium vegetable stock
- 2 cups roughly chopped Swiss chard, thoroughly washed
- 2 tablespoon white miso paste
- 1 tablespoon grated fresh ginger

**Directions:**
1. In a large saucepan over medium-high heat, bring the vegetable stock to a boil. After adding the ginger and miso paste, simmer for 5 minutes.
2. Include the whitefish and simmer for about 5 minutes, or until just cooked through. After adding the chard, simmer for three minutes, or until it has wilted. Serve right away.
**Nutritional Info:** Calories: 225; Fat: 8g; Carbs: 4g; Protein: 29g; Fiber: 0g

## Creamy Carrot Soup

Time to prepare: 15 minutes
Time to cook: 35 minutes
Servings: 4
**Ingredients:**
- 1 tablespoon olive oil
- 6 carrots, peeled & finely chopped
- 1 sweet onion, finely chopped
- 6 cups low-sodium vegetable stock
- 2 teaspoon minced garlic
- ½ cup coconut cream
- Sea salt & ground black pepper to taste

**Directions:**
1. Heat the olive oil in a large saucepan over medium heat. For approximately 3 minutes, add the onion and garlic and sauté until tender.
2. Include the vegetable stock and carrots. After bringing to a boil, reduce the heat to low and simmer the soup for about 30 minutes, or until the vegetables are tender.
3. Purée the soup in stages in a food processor until it is smooth. Add the coconut cream to the puréed soup before adding it back to the stove. Add salt and pepper, then serve.
**Nutritional Info:** Calories: 333; Fat: 22g; Carbs: 8g; Protein: 4g; Fiber: 1.3g

## Egg Drop Soup

Time to prepare: 10 minutes
Time to cook: 11 minutes
Servings: 6
**Ingredients:**
- 3 eggs
- 6 cups homemade chicken broth, divided
- 1/3 cup fresh lemon juice
- 1 tablespoon arrowroot powder (if tolerated)
- Salt & ground white pepper to taste

**Directions:**
1. Fill a soup pan with 512 cups of broth and bring to a boil over high heat. Set the heat to medium, then simmer for approximately five minutes.
2. In the meantime, combine the remaining broth, eggs, arrowroot powder, lemon juice, and white pepper in a bowl. beat until thoroughly combined.
3. While continuously stirring, add the egg mixture to your pan slowly. Simmer while stirring frequently for around 5 to 6 minutes. Serve warm.
**Nutritional Info:** Calories: 79; Fat: 3.7g; Carbs: 2.7g; Protein: 7.7g; Fiber: 0.1g

## Tomato Soup

Time to prepare: 10 minutes
Time to cook: 45 minutes
Servings: 4
**Ingredients:**
- 5 large tomatoes, peeled, seeded & chopped roughly
- 1 carrot, peeled & chopped roughly
- 3½ cups homemade vegetable broth
- ¼ cup fresh basil, chopped
- 1 tablespoon olive oil
- Salt & ground black pepper to taste

**Directions:**
1. In a large soup pan, heat the oil over medium heat. Add the carrot and cook, stirring frequently, for about 4-5 minutes.

2. Add the broth, tomatoes, basil, salt, and black pepper; stir, and bring to a boil.

3. Lower the heat to low and simmer the cover off for about 30 minutes. With the soup out of the pan, use an immersion blender to puree it. Serve warm.

**Nutritional Info:** Calories: 122; Fat: 5.2g; Carbs: 13.8g; Protein: 6.7g; Fiber: 2.8g

## Beet Soup

Time to prepare: 10 minutes
Time to cook: 5 minutes
Servings: 4

**Ingredients:**
- 2 ¼ cups beets, trimmed, peeled, and chopped
- 2 ¼ cups fat-free plain yogurt
- 2 tablespoon fresh dill
- 4 teaspoon fresh lemon juice
- Salt to taste

**Directions:**

1. Place all ingredients in a high-speed blender and mix until smooth.

2. Put the soup in a pan and heat it for 3–5 minutes, or until it is well warmed. Serve right away..

**Nutritional Info:** Calories: 87; Fat: 0.4g; Carbs: 15.9g; Protein: 6g; Fiber: 2g

## Potato Soup

Time to prepare: 15 minutes
Time to cook: 35 minutes
Servings: 6

**Ingredients:**
- 4 cups homemade chicken broth
- 4 cups potatoes, peeled & cubed
- 1 cups carrot, peeled & chopped
- ½ cup low-fat cheddar cheese
- ¼ cup fat-free plain yogurt
- 2 tablespoon olive oil
- 1 teaspoon fresh rosemary, chopped
- Salt & ground black pepper to taste

**Directions:**

1. In a large skillet over medium heat, heat the oil. Once heated, add the carrots and cook, stirring occasionally, for about 6 to 8 minutes.

2. Add the rosemary, salt, and black pepper, and cook while continuously stirring for about a minute. Let it boil before adding the potatoes and broth.

3. Cook for about 20 minutes with a partial cover. Add the yogurt and cheese, then reduce the heat to low.

4. Take out the potatoes and use a potato masher to mash half of them. Serve right away.

**Nutritional Info:** Calories: 166; Fat: 7.3g; Carbs: 19g; Protein: 6.7g; Fiber: 2.7g

## Zucchini Carrot Tomato Soup

Time to prepare: 15 minutes
Time to cook: 30 minutes
Servings: 8

**Ingredients:**
- 3 carrots, peeled & chopped
- 4 small zucchinis, peeled, seeded & chopped
- 2 tomatoes, peeled, seeded & chopped
- 8 cups vegetable broth
- Salt & ground black pepper to taste

**Directions:**

1. In your large soup pan, combine all the ingredients and heat over high heat until boiling. Set to low heat and cover partially for about 20 minutes. Remove and set aside.

2. Add the soup to the blender in batches and blend until smooth. Reintroduce the pureed mixture to the pan, reduce the heat to medium-low, and simmer for 3-5 minutes. Serve warm.

**Nutritional Info:** Calories: 63; Fat: 1.5g; Carbs: 6.3g; Protein: 6g; Fiber: 1.6g

## Yellow Squash Soup

Time to prepare: 15 minutes
Time to cook: 33 minutes

Servings: 6

**Ingredients:**

- 4 thyme sprigs
- 6 cups yellow squash, peeled, seeded & cubed
- 4 cups homemade vegetable broth
- 2 tablespoon olive oil
- 2 tablespoon fresh lemon juice
- Salt & ground black pepper to taste

**Directions:**

1. Cook the yellow squash cubes in the oil for approximately 5 minutes over medium heat in your large soup pan. Before bringing to a boil, stir in the thyme, broth, salt, and black pepper.

2. Adjust the heat to low and cook for 15 to 20 minutes with the top off. Take out and throw away the thyme sprigs. Place aside.

3. Using a large blender, add the soup in stages and process until smooth. Over medium heat, add the soup back to the same pan.

4. After adding the lemon juice, simmer for a further 2–3 minutes, or until everything is well cooked. Serve warm.

**Nutritional Info:** Calories: 85; Fat: 5.8g; Carbs: 4.5g; Protein: 4.6g; Fiber: 1.3g

## Carrot & Beet Soup

Time to prepare: 10 minutes
Time to cook: 25 minutes
Servings: 4

**Ingredients:**

- 1 carrot, peeled & sliced
- 6 oz canned cooked beets
- 4 cups low sodium vegetable broth
- Salt to taste

**Directions:**

1. Place the broth and carrot in a small saucepan over high heat and bring to a boil.

2. Adjust the heat to low and cook for about 15 minutes with the lid on. Beets should be added and cooked for 8 to 10 minutes.

3. Take out the soup pan, then use an immersion blender to puree the soup. Serve warm.

**Nutritional Info:** Calories: 40; Fat: 0.1g; Carbs: 9.7g; Protein: 0.8g; Fiber: 1.2g

## Spinach & Carrot Soup

Time to prepare: 15 minutes
Time to cook: 35 minutes
Servings: 6

**Ingredients:**

- 3 small carrots, peeled & chopped
- ¾ lb. fresh spinach, chopped
- 5 cups vegetable broth
- 2 tablespoon olive oil
- Salt & ground black pepper to taste

**Directions:**

1. In a large soup pan, heat the oil over medium heat. Cook the carrots, stirring frequently, for 8 to 10 minutes.

2. After adding the spinach, bring the broth to a boil. Cook for about 20 minutes with a partial cover.

3. Add salt and black pepper, then turn off the heat. Smoothen the soup using an immersion blender. Serve right away.

**Nutritional Info:** Calories: 125; Fat: 7.5g; Carbs: 7.1g; Protein: 8.1g; Fiber: 2.3g

## Pumpkin And Melon Soup

Time to prepare: 10 minutes
Time to cook: 30 minutes
Servings: 2

**Ingredients:**

- 1 teaspoon olive oil
- 2 cups pumpkin, peeled & diced
- 1 cup melon, peeled & diced
- 4 cups vegetable stock
- 1 teaspoon dried thyme
- Himalayan salt, to taste

**Directions:**

1. Stir the melon and pumpkin pieces while the oil in your big pot is heating. For

15 minutes, cook.

2. Include the salt, herbs, and vegetable stock. Bring everything to a boil, then simmer for an additional 12 to 15 minutes.

3. Pour the soup mixture into a blender, then blend until smooth. Serve!

**Nutritional Info:** Calories: 84; Fat: 2.6g; Carbs: 15.6g; Protein: 2.3g; Fiber: 1.7g

## Asparagus Tomato Carrots Soup

Time to prepare: 10 minutes
Time to cook: 20 minutes
Servings: 2

**Ingredients:**

- 6 asparagus stems, quartered
- 1 carrot, peeled & finely chopped
- 1 canned tomato, peeled & finely chopped
- 4 cups water
- ½ teaspoon salt
- 1 teaspoon Italian seasoning

**Directions:**

1. Place the vegetables in a soup pot or skillet and dry sauté them for one minute. Boil the water after adding it. Italian spice and salt are added.

2. For a further 15 to 20 minutes, simmer After allowing it to cool, puree it in your blender until smooth. Serve!

**Nutritional Info:** Calories: 30; Fat: 0.3g; Carbs: 6g; Protein: 2g; Fiber: 1.7g

## Squash, Pumpkin & Carrot Soup with Rice

Time to prepare: 15 minutes
Time to cook: 25 minutes
Servings: 2-3

**Ingredients:**

- 1 cup squash, peeled, deseeded & sliced
- 1 cup pumpkin, peeled, deseeded & sliced
- 1 cup carrots, peeled

- 3 cups vegetable stock
- 3 cups water
- ½ cup cooked white rice
- ½ cup lettuce
- 1 teaspoon each of dried basil, olive oil & dried thyme

**Directions:**

1. In your large pan, heat the oil, then sauté the vegetables for 5 minutes.

2. Pour the stock over the rice and add the herbs. Stirring occasionally, let it boil and simmer for about 20 minutes. Add water to make the mixture thinner.

3. Blend with an immersion blender until the mixture is smooth, then serve!

**Nutritional Info:** Calories: 70; Fat: 0.6g; Carbs: 16g; Protein: 2.3g; Fiber: 1.6g

## Creamy Tomato Lettuce Carrot Soup

Time to prepare: 10 minutes
Time to cook: 15 minutes
Servings: 2

**Ingredients:**

- 3 cups of vegetable broth
- 1 cup canned tomatoes, peeled & seeded
- 2 cups carrot, peeled and chopped
- ½ cup ricotta or cottage cheese grated
- A handful of lettuce, shredded
- 1 teaspoon olive oil
- Himalayan salt to taste

**Directions:**

1. Bring the oil in your pan to a boil before adding the fixings. 15 minutes at a simmer after adjustment.

2. Using your immersion blender, blend the ingredients until they are smooth.

**Nutritional Info:** Calories: 176; Fat: 7.6g; Carbs: 20.7g; Protein: 7.5g; Fiber: 2.4g

## Beet Sweet Potato Soup

Time to prepare: 10 minutes
Time to cook: 20-25 minutes
Servings: 2

**Ingredients:**
- 1 cup beet, peeled & diced
- 1 cup sweet potato, peeled & diced
- 3 cups vegetable stock
- 1 tablespoon olive oil
- 1 teaspoon Dijon mustard
- 1 teaspoon dried oregano
- Pinch of Himalayan salt

**Directions:**

1. Bring your pan's oil to a boil before adding the stock, vegetables, and spices.

2. Make the simmer extremely low and cook for 20 to 25 minutes. Serve after adding salt to taste.

**Nutritional Info:** Calories: 199; Fat: 7.1g; Carbs: 33.5g; Protein: 3.4g; Fiber: 2.5g

## Lettuce And Spinach Soup

Time to prepare: 10 minutes
Time to cook: 35 minutes
Servings: 2

**Ingredients:**
- 2 cups spinach fresh, chopped (if tolerated)
- 1 cup lettuce
- 3 cups vegetable stock
- 2 teaspoon olive oil
- 1 teaspoon cilantro
- 1 teaspoon whey protein
- Himalayan salt to taste

**Directions:**

1. Saute the vegetables for five minutes in a big pan. Let it boil after adding the last few ingredients.

2. Make adjustments to a simmer, then cook for about 30 minutes. Serve after blending with an immersion blender until it is smooth.

**Nutritional Info:** Calories: 61; Fat: 4.7g; Carbs: 1.9g; Protein: 3.6g; Fiber: 0.9g

## Chicken Gyro Soup

Time to prepare: 10 minutes
Time to cook: 23 minutes

Servings: 2

**Ingredients:**
- 3-4 cups broth or water
- 1 cup finely shredded chicken
- 2 canned tomatoes, peeled & finely chopped
- 1 tablespoon dried sage
- 1 teaspoon olive oil
- Salt to taste

**Directions:**

1. In your large saucepan, heat the oil, then sauté the tomatoes for two to three minutes over low heat.

3. Add 3 cups of water and bring to a boil. Add the chicken, sage, and salt after adjusting the heat to medium.

3. Simmer it for 15 to 20 minutes. Take it out, let it cool, and then serve!

**Nutritional Info:** Calories: 230; Fat: 11g; Carbs: 5.3g; Protein: 27g; Fiber: 2.1g

## Mushroom Veggie Soup

Time to prepare: 10 minutes
Time to cook: 35-40 minutes
Servings: 2

**Ingredients:**
- 1 zucchini, peeled, seeded & diced
- 3 cups water
- 2 ½ cups vegetable stock
- 2 cups mushroom, chopped
- 1 cup beet, peeled & shredded
- 1 cup lettuce, chopped
- 1 stalk of parsley, chopped
- 1 teaspoon dried oregano
- 1 teaspoon olive oil
- Himalayan salt, to taste

**Directions:**

1. For a few minutes, sauté the vegetables in olive oil in a big pot. After adding the oregano and parsley, cook for 6 to 10 minutes.

2. Add the vegetable stock and allow it to come to a boil. Stirring occasionally, cook

for 25 minutes. Utilize your immersion blender to blend until smooth. Serve!
**Nutritional Info:** Calories: 87; Fat: 3.1g; Carbs: 12.1g; Protein: 5.5g; Fiber: 2.2g

## Lettuce Cucumber Soup

Time to prepare: 10 minutes
Time to cook: 40 minutes
Servings: 2
**Ingredients:**
- 2 medium cucumbers, peeled, deseeded & diced
- 2 cups green lettuce, diced
- 3 cups vegetable stock
- 1 tablespoon olive oil
- 1 teaspoon mustard powder
- 1 teaspoon basil dried
- Himalayan salt, to taste

**Directions:**
1. In a saucepan over low heat, sauté the basil and mustard powder for 4–5 minutes.
2. After adding the water, simmer the cucumbers for 5 minutes. After adding the stock, boil the mixture for 30 minutes.

3. Pour the mixture into a blender, season with Himalayan salt, and blend until smooth. Serve hot.
**Nutritional Info:** Calories: 92; Fat: 7.2g; Carbs: 5.7g; Protein: 1.9g; Fiber: 1.9g

## Carrot Potato Soup

Time to prepare: 10 minutes
Time to cook: 0 minutes
Servings: 2
**Ingredients:**
- 2 cups carrots, peeled & sliced
- 2 cups vegetable stock
- 1 cup potato, peeled & sliced
- 1 cup non-dairy milk
- Himalayan salt to taste

**Directions:**
1. Combine all the ingredients in a pot, then cook for 25 minutes.
2. Until smooth, mix with an immersion blender. Serve

**Nutritional Info:** Calories: 174; Fat: 1.4g; Carbs: 28.6g; Protein: 6.5g; Fiber: 2.8g

# SIDES & SALADS

## Beet Salad

Time to prepare: 10 minutes
Time to cook: 0 minutes
Servings: 4
**Ingredients:**
For the Salad:
- 4 medium beets, scrubbed, roasted, peeled, &sliced
- 4 cups fresh baby spinach (if tolerated)
- 4 oz feta cheese, crumbled

For the Dressing:
- 2 tablespoon extra-virgin olive oil
- 1 tablespoon balsamic vinegar
- 1 tablespoon maple syrup
- Salt & ground black pepper to taste

**Directions:**
1. In a bowl, thoroughly combine all of the dressing's ingredients.
2. In a salad bowl, combine the beets, spinach, and dressing; toss to combine. Add feta, then plate.
**Nutritional Info:** Calories: 129; Fat: 10.2g; Carbs: 7.7g; Protein: 3.2g; Fiber: 1.3g

## Citrus Salad

Time to prepare: 10 minutes
Time to cook: 0 minutes
Servings: 6
**Ingredients:**
- 8 clementines, peeled, seeded & sliced in rounds
- 1 orange, peeled, seeded & sliced in rounds
- 2 grapefruits, peeled, seeded & sliced in rounds
- 3 tablespoon fresh lime juice
- 1 tablespoon raw honey
- 2 teaspoon lime zest

**Directions:**

1. Toss the fixings in your bowl to combine them.
2. Serve right away.
**Nutritional Info:** Calories: 92; Fat: 0.3g; Carbs: 23.4g; Protein: 1.5g; Fiber: 2.9g

## Easy Cucumber Salad

Time to prepare: 10 minutes
Time to cook: 0 minutes
Servings: 4
**Ingredients:**
- 4 medium seedless cucumbers, peeled & chopped
- ½ cup low-fat Greek yogurt
- 1½ tablespoon fresh dill, chopped
- 1 tablespoon fresh lemon juice
- Salt & ground black pepper to taste

**Directions:**
1. Toss the items in your dish to incorporate them.
2. Serve right away.
**Nutritional Info:** Calories: 71; Fat: 0.8g; Carbs: 13.8g; Protein:4g; Fiber: 1.7g

## Cucumber & Tomato Salad

Time to prepare: 10 minutes
Time to cook: 0 minutes
Servings: 5
**Ingredients:**
- 2 cups seedless cucumbers, peeled, seeded & chopped
- 2 cups tomatoes, peeled, seeded & chopped
- 2 tablespoon extra-virgin olive oil
- 2 tablespoon fresh lime juice
- Salt to taste

**Directions:**
1. Toss the fixings in your bowl to combine them.
2. Serve right away.

**Nutritional Info:** Calories: 68; Fat: 5.8g; Carbs: 04.4g; Protein: 0.9g; Fiber: 1.1g

## Parmesan Asparagus

Time to prepare: 5 minutes
Time to cook: 10 minutes
Servings: 4
**Ingredients:**
- 1 lb. asparagus tips
- ½ cup low-fat Parmesan cheese, grated freshly
- 2 tablespoon olive oil
- Salt & ground black pepper to taste

**Directions:**
1. Cook the asparagus for 10 minutes in the oil that has been heated to medium heat in your large pan.
2. Immediately serve after incorporating the parmesan, salt, and black pepper.

**Nutritional Info:** Calories: 120; Fat: 9.5g; Carbs: 3.8g; Protein: 5.2g; Fiber: 1.8g

## Parmesan Zucchini

Time to prepare: 10 minutes
Time to cook: 7 minutes
Servings: 8
**Ingredients:**
- 6 zucchinis, peeled, seeded & sliced
- ¼ cup low-fat Parmesan cheese, grated
- 3 tablespoon olive oil
- Salt & ground black pepper to taste

**Directions:**
1. In a large pan over medium-high heat, add the oil and the zucchini; cook for 5 to 6 minutes.
2. Finish by incorporating parmesan, salt, and black pepper.

**Nutritional Info:** Calories: 77; Fat: 6.1g; Carbs: 5g; Protein: 2.4g; Fiber: 1.6g

## Creamed Spinach with Tomatoes

Time to prepare: 10 minutes

Time to cook: 29 minutes
Servings: 8
**Ingredients:**
- 20 oz frozen spinach, thawed & drained
- 16 oz cottage cheese, cut into ½-inch cubes
- 2 tomatoes, peeled, seeded & chopped finely
- 1 ½ cup water, divided
- ¼ cup fat-free plain yogurt
- 2 tablespoon olive oil
- Salt to taste

**Directions:**
1. Blend the spinach, yogurt, and half a cup of water. The spinach puree dish should be set aside.
2. In your large nonstick pan, cook the tomatoes in the oil for about 3–4 minutes, breaking them up as they cook with the back of a spoon.
3. After adding the spinach puree, stir in the remaining water. Cook for three to five minutes at a medium temperature.
4. Include the cottage cheese cubes and mix well. Cook for around 10 to 15 minutes at low heat. Serve warm.

**Nutritional Info:** Calories: 109; Fat: 5g; Carbs: 7g; Protein: 10.5g; Fiber: 2g

## Lemony Green Beans

Time to prepare: 10 minutes
Time to cook: 5 minutes
Servings: 4
**Ingredients:**
- 1 lb. fresh green beans, trimmed
- 1 tablespoon olive oil
- 1 tablespoon fresh lemon juice
- 1 teaspoon lemon zest, grated
- Salt & ground black pepper to taste
- Water, as needed

**Directions:**
1. Fill a big pan with water, add a steamer basket, and bring to a boil. Place the green beans in the steamer basket and cover it

to steam them for 4-5 minutes.
2. Remove the steamer basket, then drain the green beans entirely. Toss the remaining ingredients with the green beans in a bowl to combine. Serve immediately.

**Nutritional Info:** Calories: 60; Fat: 3.5g; Carbs: 6g; Protein: 1.5g; Fiber: 2.9g

## Citrus Glazed Carrots

Time to prepare: 10 minutes
Time to cook: 14 minutes
Servings: 6
**Ingredients:**
- 1½ lb. carrots, peeled & sliced into ½-inch pieces diagonally
- ½ cup water
- 3 tablespoon fresh orange juice
- 2 tablespoon olive oil
- Salt, to taste

**Directions:**
1. Add the carrots, water, oil, and salt to a large skillet over medium heat and let it boil.
2. Adjust to low heat and simmer; cover for about 6 minutes. Add the orange juice and stir to combine.
3. Adjust to high heat and cook uncovered for about 5-8 minutes, tossing frequently. Serve immediately.

**Nutritional Info:** Calories: 86; Fat: 5g; Carbs: 10.4g; Protein: 0.9g; Fiber: 2.8g

## Braised Asparagus

Time to prepare: 5 minutes
Time to cook: 4 minutes
Servings: 2
**Ingredients:**
- 1 cup asparagus, trimmed
- ½ cup chicken bone broth
- 1 tablespoon olive oil
- 1 (½-inch) lemon peel

**Directions:**

1. Add the asparagus and simmer it for 3 to 4 minutes with the lid off. Serve after discarding the lemon peel. heat 1. Blend the spinach, yogurt, and 1/2 cup of water in a blender. Set aside the dish with the spinach purée.
2. Cook the tomatoes in the oil in a big nonstick skillet for about 3–4 minutes, breaking them up along the way with the back of a spoon. 3. Stir in the remaining water after adding the spinach puree. Cook at a medium temperature for three to five minutes.

**Nutritional Info:** Calories: 94; Fat: 7.8g; Carbs: 3.9g; Protein: 3.7g; Fiber: 2.2g

## Mexican Avocado Salad

Time to prepare: 10 minutes
Time to cook: 15 minutes
Servings: 4
**Ingredients:**
- 4 large fresh avocados, roughly chopped
- 1 beefsteak tomato, peeled, seeded & chopped
- 2 to 3 limes, zest, and juice
- ½ cup sliced red onion (if tolerated)
- ¼ cup chopped cilantro
- 1 tablespoon extra-virgin olive oil
- ½ teaspoon salt
- ¼ teaspoon freshly ground pepper

**Directions:**
1. In a large bowl, mix the onion, avocados, tomato, and cilantro.
2. Add salt and pepper to taste, then top with lime juice, olive oil, and zest. Serve!

**Nutritional Info:** Calories: 277; Fat: 24.6g; Carbs: 16.8g; Protein: 3.3g; Fiber: 2.4g

## Baked Butternut Squash

Time to prepare: 10 minutes
Time to cook: 45 minutes
Servings: 6

**Ingredients:**
- 5 cups butternut squash, peeled, seeded & cubed
- 2 tablespoon olive oil
- Salt to taste

**Directions:**
1. Set the oven's temperature to 425°F and divide the foil across two baking pans.
2. Combine all the ingredients in a large dish and toss to evenly coat
3. Place the squash pieces in a single layer on the preheated baking pans. For around 40 to 45 minutes, roast. Serve warm.

**Nutritional Info:** Calories: 93; Fat: 4.8g; Carbs: 13.6g; Protein: 1.2g; Fiber: 2.3g

## Spinach In Yogurt Sauce

Time to prepare: 10 minutes
Time to cook: 7 minutes
Servings: 4

**Ingredients:**
- 2 (10-oz.) packages of frozen spinach, thawed & squeezed dry
- ½ cup fat-free plain yogurt
- 2 tablespoon olive oil
- 1 teaspoon fresh lemon juice
- Salt & ground black pepper to taste

**Directions:**
1. In the pan, heat the oil to medium heat before adding the spinach and cooking it for one to two minutes. Yogurt is added and cooked for three to five minutes.
2. Add the lemon juice, salt, and black pepper, then turn off the heat. Serve right away.

**Nutritional Info:** Calories: 85; Fat: 6.1g; Carbs: 5.8g; Protein: 4.3g; Fiber: 2.3g

## Cucumber Peach Salad

Time to prepare: 30 minutes
Time to cook: 0 minutes
Servings: 4

**Ingredients:**

- 2 large avocados, pitted & diced
- 1 peach, peeled, pitted & diced
- 1 gala pear, peeled, cored & diced
- 1 English cucumber, peeled, seeded & chopped
- 1 cup cantaloupe, peeled, seeded & chopped
- 1 shallot, chopped finely (if tolerated)
- ¼ cup fresh lime juice
- ¼ cup fresh mint, chopped
- 2 Large lettuce leaves

**Directions:**
1. Bring the oil in the pan to medium heat, add the spinach, and cook for 1–2 minutes. After adding the sugar, the yogurt is heated for three to five minutes.
2. After adding the salt, black pepper, and lemon juice, turn off the heat. Serve immediately.

**Nutritional Info:** Calories: 182; Fat: 11g; Carbs: 23g; Protein: 6g; Fiber: 0.4g

## Sweet Poppy Seed Salad

Time to prepare: 10 minutes
Time to cook: 0 minutes
Servings: 6

**Ingredients:**
- 1/3 cup distilled white vinegar
- ½ cup olive oil
- ¼ cup maple syrup
- ¼ cup pumpkin puree
- 1/8 teaspoon salt
- ½ teaspoon minced garlic
- 2 teaspoon poppy seeds
- 1 lb. lettuce of choice

**Directions:**
1. Add the spinach to the pan and cook for 1–2 minutes with the oil over medium heat. The yogurt is cooked for three to five minutes after the sugar has been added.
2. Switch off the heat after adding the salt, black pepper, and lemon juice. Serve right away.

**Nutritional Info:** Calories: 321; Fat: 28g; Carbs: 17g; Protein: 2g; Fiber: 2g;

## Watermelon-Tomato Salad

Time to prepare: 10 minutes
Time to cook: 0 minutes
Servings: 4

**Ingredients:**
- 3 cups heirloom tomato wedges, peeled, seeded & sliced
- 3 cups seedless watermelon, cut into 1-inch cubes
- 3 cups trimmed watercress (if tolerated)
- 6 tablespoon feta cheese crumbles
- 2 tablespoon extra-virgin olive oil
- 2 tablespoon chopped fresh basil (if tolerated)
- 1½ tablespoon sherry vinegar
- Pinch of salt & ground black pepper

**Directions:**
1. In a small bowl, combine the oil, vinegar, salt, and pepper.
2. Combine the tomatoes, watermelon, watercress, and basil in a big bowl.
3. Drizzle the salad with the dressing and toss to coat. Serve after adding the feta cheese on top.

**Nutritional Info:** Calories: 165; Fat: 11g; Carbs: 17g; Protein: 5g; Fiber: 2g

## Cinnamon Peaches & Apple

Time to prepare: 10 minutes
Time to cook: 40 minutes
Servings: 6

**Ingredients:**

- 4 peaches, skin removed & thinly sliced
- 1 lb. apple, peeled, cored & sliced
- 1 cup honey or maple syrup
- 1 teaspoon cinnamon powder
- 1 teaspoon vanilla extract

**Directions:**

1. Combine the oil, vinegar, salt, and pepper in a small bowl.
2. In a large bowl, mix the tomatoes, watermelon, watercress, and basil.
3. Pour the dressing over the salad and toss to combine. Serve after topping with feta cheese.

**Nutritional Info:** Calories: 178; Fat: 4g; Carbs: 7g; Protein: 27g; Fiber: 2g

## Sweet Potato Chips with Avocado Smash

Time to prepare: 10 minutes
Time to cook: 30 minutes
Servings: 8

**Ingredients:**

- 2 peeled sweet potatoes, cut into thin slices
- 1 avocado, pitted & sliced
- 1/4 cup coriander, chopped
- 1/4 cup lime juice
- 1 teaspoon sumac
- Salt & pepper to taste
- Cooking spray

**Directions:**

1. Preheat the oven to 400 degrees Fahrenheit and oil 2 baking sheets.
2. Set the prepared tray with the sweet potatoes on it. After spraying, bake the slices for 20 minutes. After flipping, spraying with oil, and baking for ten minutes,
3. Mash the avocado in a bowl with the sumac, coriander, lime juice, and salt. Along with the potato chips, serve the avocado mixture.

**Nutritional Info:** Calories 45; Fat 3g; Carbs 14g; Protein 3g; Fiber 2g

## Vegetable Fritters

Time to prepare: 15 minutes
Time to cook: 3 minutes
Servings: 4

**Ingredients:**

- 2 large eggs
- 1 large carrot, peeled & spiralized
- 1 zucchini, peeled, seeded & spiralized
- 1 russet potato, peeled & sliced into thin strips
- 1 medium onion, halved & thinly sliced
- ½ cup extra-virgin olive oil
- 2 teaspoon sea salt
- Freshly ground black pepper to taste

**Directions:**

1. Combine the onion, potato, carrot, and zucchini in a colander and season with salt. Give the vegetables about 15 minutes to stand. Use a paper towel to dry.
2. Whip the eggs and add pepper to a separate bowl. After adding the vegetables, stir to coat them.
3. Add a little oil to a big pan that is already hot over medium-high heat.
4. Form thin patties by scooping about 14 cups of the vegetable mixture at a time. They should be dropped into the hot pan and fried for two to three minutes, or until golden brown.
5. Rotate, then repeat on the opposite

side. Serve after transferring to a plate lined with paper towels.
**Nutritional Info:** Calories: 131; Fat: 12g; Carbs: 5g; Protein: 2g; Fiber: 1g

## Applesauce

Time to prepare: 10 minutes
Time to cook: 30 minutes
Servings: 4
**Ingredients:**
- 6 organic apples, peeled, cored, & cubed
- ½ cup boiling water
- ½ teaspoon cinnamon powder
- 4 tablespoon honey
- 2 tablespoon fresh lemon juice
- ¼ teaspoon salt

**Directions:**
1. Boiling water, lemon juice, cinnamon, honey, and salt should all be added to your big saucepan along with the apples to simmer them until they are tender. Get rid of the heat.
2. In a blender, thoroughly combine the ingredients in this combination. Put the applesauce in a container or jar of your choice. Serve hot or chilly.
**Nutritional Info:** Calories: 51; Fat: 3g; Carbs: 4g; Protein: 2g; Fiber: 2g

## Cinnamon Pear Chips

Time to prepare: 10 minutes
Time to cook: 3 hours
Servings: 4
**Ingredients:**
- 4 pears, peeled, cored & cut into 1/8-inch slices
- 1 teaspoon ground cinnamon

**Directions:**
1. Preheat the oven to 200 degrees Fahrenheit, then line a baking sheet with parchment paper.
2. In a bowl, combine the pears and cinnamon and toss to combine.

3. Arrange the pears on the preheated baking sheet in a single layer. Cook the pears for 2 to 3 hours, or until they are dry. Serve!
**Nutritional Info:** Calories: 83; Fat: 0g; Carbs: 19g; Protein: 1g; Fiber: 1g

## Avocado Dip

Time to prepare: 10 minutes
Time to cook: 0 minutes
Servings: 4
**Ingredients:**
- 6 avocados, peeled & pitted
- ½ tablespoon extra-virgin olive oil
- ¼ cup chopped fresh cilantro
- 2 tablespoon fresh lime juice
- 1 teaspoon fresh lemon juice
- ½ teaspoon salt

**Directions:**
1. In a bowl, combine all the ingredients and stir until well combined.
2. Dish out and savor!
**Nutritional Info:** Calories: 75; Fat: 1.7g; Carbs: 0.1g; Protein: 13.4g; Fiber: 3.7g

## Egg Potato Bites

Time to prepare: 10 minutes
Time to cook: 25 minutes
Servings: 12 bites
**Ingredients:**
- 8 eggs
- 8 oz cooked & peeled potato, chopped
- 1 cup cottage cheese, pureed
- 2 oz Swiss cheese
- Salt, to taste
- Cooking spray

**Directions:**
1. Oil-spray a 12-cup muffin tin and preheat the oven to 325°F.
2. Combine the eggs, potatoes, salt, and cottage cheese in a bowl. Add the mixture to the cups 30 minutes later, top with cheese, and bake. Serve!
**Nutritional Info:** Calories 90; Fat 4g; Carbs 3g; Protein 8g; Fiber 1g

## Potato Sticks

Time to prepare: 15 minutes
Time to cook: 10 minutes
Servings: 2
**Ingredients:**
- 1 large russet potato, peeled & cut into sticks
- 10 curry leaves
- 1 tablespoon olive oil
- ¼ teaspoon ground turmeric
- Salt, to taste

**Directions:**
1. Spread parchment paper across 2 baking sheets.
2. Place all the fixings in your bowl and toss to evenly coat. Place the potatoes in a single layer on your baking sheets.
3. After 10 minutes of baking in your preheated oven, serve right away.

**Nutritional Info:** Calories: 187; Fat: 9g; Carbs: 26g; Protein: 14g; Fiber: 1g

## Beet Chips

Time to prepare: 15 minutes
Time to cook: 20 minutes
Servings: 2
**Ingredients:**
- 1 beetroot, trimmed, peeled & sliced thinly
- 1 teaspoon garlic, minced
- 2 teaspoon olive oil
- Salt, to taste

**Directions:**
1. In a big bowl, combine all the fixings and toss to thoroughly coat. Spread the mixture out evenly on your baking sheet.
2. Bake for 20 minutes, flipping once, in your preheated oven. Serve right away.

**Nutritional Info:** Calories: 80; Fat: 4.5g; Carbs: 6g; Protein: 3g; Fiber: 2g

## Homemade Hummus

Time to prepare: 10 minutes

Time to cook: 60 minutes
Servings: 4
**Ingredients:**
- ¼-lb dried chickpeas, soaked in water for a night
- 1 ½ tablespoon tahini
- 1 tablespoon lemon juice
- 2 tablespoon extra-virgin olive oil
- ¼ teaspoon cumin powder
- ½ teaspoon salt
- 1 tablespoon water

**Directions:**
1. Boil your chickpeas for approximately an hour in a big pot of water over medium heat. Drain well, then let it cool.
2. Add it to the blender along with 1 tablespoon of olive oil, salt, tahini, lemon juice, and cumin powder. Blend the hummus until it has a uniformly soft and creamy texture.
3. Add 1 tablespoon of extra-virgin olive oil, and serve!

**Nutritional Info:** Calories: 207; Fat: 16g; Carbs: 5g; Protein: 12g; Fiber: 1g

## Baked Apricots with Honey

Time to prepare: 10 minutes
Time to cook: 15 minutes
Servings: 4
**Ingredients:**
- 4 ripe apricots, halved & pitted
- ¼ cup raw honey
- ¼ teaspoon ground ginger
- ¼ teaspoon ground nutmeg
- Cooking spray

**Directions:**
1. Preheat the oven to 400°F and spray cooking spray on a sizable baking pan.
2. Place the apricots on the prepared pan in a single layer and cut the sides up. Honey should be drizzled over the apricots before adding the ginger and nutmeg.
3. Bake the apricots for 12 to 15 minutes, or until they are soft. Serve!

**Nutritional Info:** Calories: 121; Fat: 4g; Carbs: 23g; Protein: 2g; Fiber: 2g

## Pear And Apple Crisps

Time to prepare: 10 minutes
Time to cook: 30 minutes
Servings: 2
**Ingredients:**
- 1 large apple, peeled, cored & thinly sliced
- 1 large pear, peeled, cored & thinly sliced
- 1 tablespoon olive oil
- 1 teaspoon cinnamon
- Himalayan salt to taste

**Directions:**
1. Preheat the oven to 410 degrees Fahrenheit and foil a baking sheet.
2. Arrange the fruit on the baking sheet, drizzle some oil over it, and sprinkle some cinnamon on top.
3. Bake it for 30 minutes or until it's tender, then let it cool before serving!
**Nutritional Info:** Calories: 108; Fat: 0.1g; Carbs: 14g; Protein: 0.3g; Fiber: 1.4g

## Peach And Cream

Time to prepare: 10 minutes
Time to cook: 0 minutes
Servings: 2
**Ingredients:**
- ½ cup fat-free cream
- ¼ cup coconut water
- 1 cup canned peaches
- ½ tablespoon honey
- A pinch of Himalayan salt

**Directions:**
1. In a blender, combine the cream, coconut water, honey, and Himalayan salt until thoroughly combined.
2. Spoon the mixture into a bowl, then add the peaches on top.
**Nutritional Info:** Calories: 108; Fat: 2.1g; Carbs: 24.4g; Protein: 1g; Fiber: 1.3g

## Herby Cheese Biscuits

Time to prepare: 10 minutes
Time to cook: 15-20 minutes
Servings: 6-8 biscuits
**Ingredients:**
- 1 cup all-purpose flour
- ¼ teaspoon salt
- 6 tablespoon cold butter
- ¼ cup buttermilk
- ½ tablespoon dried parsley
- ½ tablespoon baking powder
- ¼ teaspoon garlic powder
- ½ cup parmesan cheese, grated
- ½ tablespoon dried thyme

**Directions:**
1. Preheat the oven to 400 degrees Fahrenheit and line a baking sheet with parchment paper.
2. In a bowl, combine the flour, salt, baking powder, and garlic powder. To make a coarse dough, combine the cold butter and add it.
3. After thoroughly combining the cheese and herbs, add the buttermilk gradually. Mix to create a dough that is neither sticky nor dry.
4. Scoop 1/4 cup of dough per biscuit into a baking pan that has been greased. Bake for 15 to 20 minutes, or until the bottom and sides are golden..
**Nutritional Info:** Calories: 184; Fat: 10.2g; Carbs: 8.3g; Protein: 5g; Fiber: 0.6g

## Low-Fiber Apple Butter

Time to prepare: 10 minutes
Time to cook: 35 minutes
Servings: 1 small jar
**Ingredients:**
- 2 cups apples, peeled, cored & grated
- 3 tablespoon maple syrup
- 1/3 cup water
- 1 tablespoon apple cider vinegar
- A pinch of cinnamon

- A pinch of salt

**Directions:**

1. Fill a pan with a wide bottom with water and add the apples. Add the vinegar, maple syrup, and salt.
2. Set it to a vigorous boil. Set the temperature to a simmer and cook for 15 minutes. To keep it from burning, stir it frequently.
3. Remove, let cool, and puree in your blender. Cook once more for 20 to 25 minutes at medium heat.
4. Add a pinch of cinnamon for flavor and thoroughly stir. Serve right away or put it in a jar for later.

**Nutritional Info:** Calories: 56; Fat: 0g; Carbs: 9.4g; Protein: 1g; Fiber: 0.5g

## Rice Flakes Protein Bar

Time to prepare: 10 minutes + chilling time
Time to cook: 0 minutes
Servings: 8-10 bars

**Ingredients:**

- ¾ cup smooth peanut butter
- 2 tablespoon maple syrup
- ¼ cup canned nectarines, finely chopped
- ¼ cup protein powder
- ½ cup toasted rice or corn flakes
- ¼ teaspoon salt

**Directions:**

1. In a frying pan over low heat, toast the rice flakes for 5 minutes. Set aside for cooling.
2. In a bowl, mix the flakes and other ingredients after crushing them. To make a dough, thoroughly combine all of the ingredients.
3. Spread into a 4 x 4 pan that has been parchment paper-lined. Allow it to chill for two to three hours. Take it out, slice it into bars, and serve!

**Nutritional Info:** Calories: 128; Fat: 5.3g; Carbs: 15.6g; Protein: 4.7g; Fiber: 1g

## Low-Fiber Ketchup

Time to prepare: 10 minutes
Time to cook: 10 minutes
Servings: 2 cups

**Ingredients:**

- 2 medium carrots, peeled & cut into quarters
- 2 cups tomato, peeled, seeded & cut into small pieces
- ¼ cup water
- 1 tablespoon apple cider vinegar
- 1 teaspoon extra virgin olive oil
- ½ teaspoon honey
- Pink Himalayan salt, to taste

**Directions:**

1. In a blender, puree everything but the oil until smooth.
2. Add the puree mixture after heating the oil in your saucepan. Cook until soft for 10 to 15 minutes; if necessary, add more water. Serve!

**Nutritional Info:** Calories: 25; Fat: 0.2g; Carbs: 6.2g; Protein: 0.4g; Fiber: 0.9g

## Sweet Dill Dip

Time to prepare: 10 minutes
Time to cook: 0 minutes
Servings: ½ cup

**Ingredients:**

- ½ cup organic plain yogurt
- A handful of fresh dill leaves, finely chopped
- 1 teaspoon honey

**Directions:**

1. Use a blender to thoroughly combine all the ingredients.
2. Use as a dip with whatever you choose, or serve with cracked wheat and peeled fruit.

**Nutritional Info:** Calories: 25; Fat: 1g; Carbs: 3g; Protein: 1.2g; Fiber: 0g

## Peanut Butter Dill Dressing

Time to prepare: 10 minutes
Time to cook: 0 minutes
Servings: ¼ cup
**Ingredients:**
- ¼ cup smooth peanut butter
- 3 tablespoon warm water
- A sprig of dill leaves
- A pinch of pink Himalayan salt

**Directions:**
1. Use a blender to thoroughly combine all the ingredients.
2. Consume now or keep in the fridge for later

**Nutritional Info:** Calories: 93; Fat: 5.3g; Carbs: 7.9g; Protein: 2.3g; Fiber: 0.6g

## Cheesy Dill Dressing

Time to prepare: 10 minutes
Time to cook: 0 minutes
Servings: 2-3
**Ingredients:**
- ½ cup parmesan
- ¼ cup dill, chopped
- 1 tablespoon soy sauce
- 1 cup water

**Directions:**
1. Use a blender to thoroughly combine all the ingredients.
2. Consume now or keep in the fridge for later.

**Nutritional Info:** Calories: 56; Fat: 0.7g; Carbs: 6.4g; Protein: 6g; Fiber: 0.2g.

## Strawberry Gummies

Time to prepare: 5 minutes + cooling time
Time to cook: 20 minutes
Servings: 4
**Ingredients:**
- 1 cup strawberries, hulled, chopped
- ¾ cup water
- 2 tablespoon gelatin

**Directions:**
1. In a large saucepan over high heat, bring the water and berries to a boil. As soon as the mixture starts to boil, remove it from the heat.
2. Add to your blender and process until smooth. Remix after adding the gelatin. Fill a silicone mold for gummy bears with your mixture.
3. Put on a tray and refrigerate for about 4 hours to set. Serve!

**Nutritional Info:** Calories: 24; Fat: 0.1g; Carbs: 2.9g; Protein: 3.2g; Fiber: 0.7g

## Fruity Jell-O Stars

Time to prepare: 15 minutes + cooling time
Time to cook: 0 minutes
Servings: 4
**Ingredients:**
- 1 tablespoon gelatin, powdered
- ¾ cup boiling water
- 3 ½ cups canned fruit
- 1 tablespoon honey
- 1 teaspoon lemon juice

**Directions:**
1. In a blender, combine all the ingredients except the gelatin. Remix after adding the gelatin.
2. Spoon the mixture into a silicone gummy mold. Refrigerate for about 4 hours to set on your tray. Serve!

**Nutritional Info:** Calories: 50; Fat: 0g; Carbs: 11.8g; Protein: 1.8g; Fiber: 0.9g

## Cranberry Kombucha Jell-O

Time to prepare: 5 minutes + chilling time
Time to cook: 0 minutes
Servings: 6
**Ingredients:**
- ¼ cup water, at room temperature
- ¼ cup hot water
- 1 tablespoon gelatin

- 1 cup unsweetened cranberry kombucha

**Directions:**
1. Combine the gelatin and room-temperature water in your bowl, stirring until fully dissolved.
2. Stir in hot water, then leave it to rest for about 2 minutes. Add in the kombucha and stir until combined.
3. Transfer to your containers, then place on a tray in the refrigerator to set for about 4 hours. Serve!

**Nutritional Info:** Calories: 15; Fat: 0g; Carbs: 0.9g; Protein: 0g; Fiber: 0g

## Apple Cider Muffins

Time to prepare: 15 minutes
Time to cook: 14 minutes
Servings: 12 muffins
**Ingredients:**
- 2 cups all-purpose flour
- ½ cup stevia
- 1 teaspoon baking soda
- 1 teaspoon baking powder
- 1 teaspoon pumpkin pie spice
- ¼ teaspoon table salt
- 1 cup apple cider
- 2 tablespoon avocado oil
- ¼ cup no-added-sugar applesauce
- ½ cup unsweetened nondairy milk
- 1 teaspoon pure vanilla extract
- Nonstick cooking spray

**Directions:**
1. Spray a muffin tin with cooking spray and preheat the oven to 350°F. Place aside.
2. In a medium bowl, stir together the flour, stevia, baking soda, baking powder, pumpkin pie spice, and salt.
3. In a separate dish, combine the apple cider, oil, applesauce, milk, and vanilla. Fold in the remaining wet components after combining the dry ingredients with half of the wet ones.

4. Fill each muffin pan to approximately 3/4 full. Bake for 12 to 14 minutes, or until golden brown on top. After one minute of cooling in the pan, place the muffins on a wire rack.

**Nutritional Info:** Calories: 168; Fat: 3g; Carbs: 33g; Protein: 2g; Fiber: 1g

## Plum & Nectarine Pudding

Time to prepare: 15 minutes + chilling time
Time to cook: 0 minutes
Servings: 5
**Ingredients:**
- 1 large nectarine, peeled, seeded & sliced
- 2 small plums, peeled & seeded
- 2 tablespoon gelatin
- 1 ½ cup water, room temperature
- 2 cups boiling water
- 2 teaspoon lemon juice
- 1/8 cup honey
- 1 teaspoon vanilla
- 1/2 teaspoon sea salt

**Directions:**
1. Blend the fruits, water at room temperature, lemon juice, and vanilla until smooth. A filter is passed through a strainer with a fine mesh.
2. Mix the fruit mixture with the gelatin while stirring to completely dissolve it. Add boiling water, stir, and then let sit for approximately two minutes.
3. Add the last of the ingredients and mix to blend.
4. Transfer to your containers, then put on a tray and chill for around 4 hours to set. Serve!

**Nutritional Info:** Calories: 99; Fat: 0.1g; Carbs: 23g; Protein: 2.8g; Fiber: 0.7g

## Rice Pudding

Time to prepare: 5 minutes
Time to cook: 5 minutes

Servings: 4

**Ingredients:**

- 1 cup unsweetened nondairy milk
- 2 tablespoon pure maple syrup
- 1 tablespoon chia seeds
- 1 teaspoon ground cinnamon
- Pinch of salt
- 2 cups cooked jasmine rice

**Directions:**

1. In a small saucepan over medium-high heat, combine the salt, cinnamon, milk, maple syrup, and chia seeds.

2. Within five minutes, bring the mixture to a simmer. After that, turn off the heat and toss in the cooked rice. Give it a cover and two minutes to rest. Serve hot or cold.

**Nutritional Info:** Calories: 227; Fat: 3g; Carbs: 47g; Protein: 5g; Fiber: 2g

## Chocolate English Custard

Time to prepare: 10 minutes + chilling time

Time to cook: 10 minutes

Servings: 2

**Ingredients:**

- 1½ tablespoon tapioca starch
- 1 egg
- 1 tablespoon pure maple syrup
- ¾ cup almond milk
- 1 tablespoon water
- 1½ tablespoon cocoa powder

**Directions:**

1. Place all the ingredients in a pot and whisk to eliminate any lumps. Put the pan on the burner and bring to a boil while stirring continuously.

2. As soon as the mixture thickens, turn off the heat. Pour the mixture into ramekins, then chill for three hours before serving.

**Nutritional Info:** Calories: 122; Fat: 3.6g; Carbs: 20.5g; Protein: 3.9g; Fiber: 1.6g

## Lemon Bars

Time to prepare: 15 minutes

Time to cook: 30 minutes

Servings: 12 bars

**Ingredients:**

- 2 cups all-purpose flour
- 1/2 cup powdered stevia
- 2 sticks of butter, each cut into 5 pieces
- 2 cups granulated stevia
- 4 eggs, beaten
- 2/3 cup lemon juice
- 1 tablespoon lemon zest
- 1-1/2 tablespoon cornstarch (if tolerated)
- 1 teaspoon baking powder
- 1/4 teaspoon salt

**Directions:**

1. Oven temperature: 300 degrees Fahrenheit.

2. Before incorporating the flour, pulse the butter and stevia powder in a food processor. The crust should cover the whole bottom of a glass baking dish measuring 9 by 13 inches in size.

3. Take the crust out of the oven and set it aside after 25 minutes of baking.

4. In a bowl, mash together the stevia, eggs, cornstarch, baking soda, and salt. The crust should be covered with the filling.

5. Bake the bars at 350 degrees Fahrenheit for 28 to 30 minutes, or until the filling is set. Serve!

**Nutritional Info:** Calories: 311; Fat: 16.8g; Carbs: 39.6g; Protein: 2.1g; Fiber: 0.0g

## Lemon Gelatin

Time to prepare: 10 minutes + chilling time

Time to cook: 0 minutes

Servings: 2

**Ingredients:**

- 3 tablespoon powdered gelatin
- 1½ cup stevia
- 1 1/2 cups boiling water
- 3 cups cold water
- 1 1/8 cups lemon juice
- 1/2 teaspoon lemon zest

**Directions:**
1. Stir the gelatin and water together until completely dissolved. Add hot water, stir, and then let sit for about two minutes.
2. Stir to combine after adding all the additional fixings.
3. Transfer to your containers, then put on a tray and chill for about 4 hours to set. Serve!

**Nutritional Info:** Calories: 66; Fat: 0.3g; Carbs: 135.6g; Protein: 9.4g; Fiber: 0.4g

## Sugar–Free Cinnamon Jelly

Time to prepare: 10 minutes + chilling time
Time to cook: 0 minutes
Servings: 2

**Ingredients:**
- 1 cup hot herbal tea
- 1 cup room temperature water
- 2 teaspoon gelatin
- 1/3 cup stevia

**Directions:**
1. Stir your gelatin and water together until completely dissolved. Add the herbal tea, stir, and let sit for about two minutes.
2. Include the gelatin and stir everything together. Transfer to your containers, then put on a tray and chill for about 4 hours to set. Serve!

**Nutritional Info:** Calories: 113; Fat: 0g; Carbs: 28.4g; Protein: 2.2g; Fiber: 0g

## Grapefruit Gelatin

Time to prepare: 10 minutes + chilling time
Time to cook: 3-5 minutes
Servings: 4

**Ingredients:**
- 1 tablespoon grass-fed gelatin powder
- 1¼ cup fresh grapefruit juice
- ¾ cup cold water, divided
- ¼ cup raw honey
- pinch of sea salt

**Directions:**
1. Soak the gelatin in 1/4 cup of cold water in a bowl. Place aside.
2. In your small saucepan, combine the remaining water and honey and heat to a boil. Three minutes should be sufficient for the honey to completely dissolve.
3. Take out and mix in the soaked gelatin until it completely dissolves. Place aside.
4. Add the salt and grapefruit juice after cooling. When ready, place the mixture in your serving bowls and chill for around 4 hours.

**Nutritional Info:** Calories: 94; Fat: 0.1g; Carbs: 23.3g; Protein: 2g; Fiber: 0g

## Tangerine Gelatin

Time to prepare: 10 minutes
Time to cook: 0 minutes
Servings: 4

**Ingredients:**
- 1 tablespoon Grass-fed tangerine gelatin powder
- 2 ¼ cups Boiling water

**Directions:**
1. In a large dish, combine the gelatin and the boiling water. Stir until the gelatin is thoroughly dissolved.
2. Before serving, divide the mixture into serving dishes and chill until totally set.

**Nutritional Info:** Calories: 13; Fat: 0g; Carbs: 0.4g; Protein: 2.8g; Fiber: 0g

## Grape Gelatin

Time to prepare: 10 minutes + chilling time
Time to cook: 0 minutes
Servings: 8

**Ingredients:**

- 1 tablespoon grass-fed gelatin powder
- ¼ cup hot water
- ¼ cup cold water
- 1 cup fresh grape juice

**Directions:**

1. Place the gelatin in a basin and cover with cold water. Wait for roughly five minutes.

2. Stir thoroughly after adding the hot water. Wait for around one or two minutes. Blend in the grape juice after adding it.

3. Distribute into serving dishes and chill until totally set before using.

**Nutritional Info:** Calories: 15; Fat: 0g; Carbs: 2.8g; Protein: 0.9g; Fiber: 0g

## Apple Gelatin

Time to prepare: 10 minutes + chilling time
Time to cook: 0 minutes
Servings: 6

**Ingredients:**

- 1 tablespoon grass-fed gelatin powder
- ¼ cup boiling water
- 1 ¾ cup warm fresh apple juice
- 1-2 drops of fresh lemon juice

**Directions:**

1. Gelatin powder should be added to a medium basin. Just enough warm apple juice should be added to completely cover the gelatin.

2. Set aside within 2 to 3 minutes, or until a thick syrup develops. When the gelatin is all dissolved, add the boiling water and whisk until it is.

3. Continue stirring after adding the remaining apple juice and lemon juice.

4. Place the mixture in a baking dish lined with parchment paper and chill for two hours, or until the top is solid, before serving.

**Nutritional Info:** Calories: 37; Fat: 0.1g; Carbs: 8.2g; Protein: 1.1g; Fiber: 0.2g

## Peach Gelatin

Time to prepare: 10 minutes + chilling time
Time to cook: 5 minutes
Servings: 10

**Ingredients:**

- 2 tablespoon grass-fed gelatin powder
- 2 tablespoon honey
- 4 ½ cups fresh peach juice, divided

**Directions:**

1. Soak the gelatin in 1/2 cup of juice in a dish. Wait for roughly five minutes.

2. Place the leftover liquid in a medium skillet over medium heat and bring to a moderate boil. Remove, then incorporate honey.

3. After adding it, whisk the gelatin mixture until it dissolves. Before serving, place the mixture in a sizable baking dish and chill until fully set.

**Nutritional Info:** Calories: 66; Fat: 0g; Carbs: 15.5g; Protein: 1.2g; Fiber: 0g

## Cinnamon Gelatin

Time to prepare: 10 minutes
Time to cook: 5 minutes
Servings: 2

**Ingredients:**

- 1 cup of filtered water
- 1 cinnamon stick
- 2 teaspoon grass-fed gelatin powder
- 2 tablespoon honey

**Directions:**

1. Add the water to a small pan and bring it to a boil over medium heat. Turn off the heat after incorporating the cinnamon stick.

2. Cover the pan right away and steep for 3 minutes. Blend in the gelatin after adding it.

3. Spoon the mixture into your baking dish, and then let it sit there to cool for around two hours. set in the refrigerator before serving.

**Nutritional Info:** Calories: 76; Fat: 0g; Carbs: 17.3g; Protein: 3.7g; Fiber: 0g

## Cinnamon Stuffed Peaches

Time to prepare: 10 minutes
Time to cook: 15 minutes
Servings: 4
**Ingredients:**
- 4 peaches, peeled, pitted, & halved
- 2 tablespoon ricotta cheese
- 2 tablespoon raw honey
- ¾ cup water
- ½ teaspoon vanilla extract
- ¾ teaspoon ground cinnamon
- ¾ teaspoon saffron

**Directions:**
1. Fill the pot with water, then wait for it to boil. Add the liquid honey, saffron, ground cinnamon, and vanilla essence. Until the honey has melted, simmer the liquid.
2. Remove and stir the peach halves into the heated honey mixture.
3. In the meanwhile, combine the vanilla essence and ricotta cheese in a basin.
4. Take the peaches out of the liquid honey and place them on the platter. Four peach halves should be filled with ricotta filling before the remaining four halves are placed on top.
5. Lightly sprinkle the liquid honey mixture over the prepared dessert.

**Nutritional Info:** Calories: 104; Fat: 2.4g; Carbs: 19.9g; Protein: 2.26g; Fiber: 2.3g

## Rustic Carrot Cake

Time to prepare: 15 minutes
Time to cook: 35 minutes
Servings: 24 slices
**Ingredients:**
- 2 cups gluten-free all-purpose flour
- 2 teaspoon baking powder
- 1 teaspoon baking soda
- 1 cup vegetable oil
- 4 large eggs
- 2 teaspoon cinnamon
- 1 teaspoon vanilla extract
- 1 lb. carrots, peeled & grated
- ¾ cup raisins
- 1 teaspoon salt
- ¾ cup stevia

**Directions:**
1. Preheat the oven to 350 degrees Fahrenheit. Grease or line a cake pan with parchment paper.
2. In a bowl, stir together the flour, baking powder, baking soda, and salt. Place aside.
3. Combine the remaining ingredients in another bowl. Fold the ingredients together after adding the wet components to the dry ones.
4. After adding the mixture to the cake pan, bake it for 35 minutes. Let it cool before serving.
5. Let the cake pan cool completely before removing it.

**Nutritional Info:** Calories: 173; Fat: 11.2g; Carbs: 19.2g; Protein: 1.7g; Fiber: 1.3g

## Lemon Cake

Time to prepare: 15 minutes
Time to cook: 45 minutes
Servings: 10
**Ingredients:**
- 1 cup olive oil
- 2 cups refined flour
- 4 tablespoon baking powder
- 4 eggs
- 4 tablespoon almond milk
- Zest from 1 lemon, grated
- 1 cup stevia

**Directions:**
1. Preheat the oven to 350 degrees Fahrenheit and butter a baking dish.
2. In a large bowl, mix the olive oil, flour, baking powder, eggs, almond milk, stevia, and lemon zest.
3. Pour the batter into the baking dish.

Aluminum foil should be used to cover the pan. Bake for 45 minutes. Let it cool before serving.

**Nutritional Info:** Calories: 508; Fat: 28.6g; Carbs: 61g; Protein: 4.3g; Fiber: 0.1g

## Vanilla Sponge Cake

Time to prepare: 15 minutes
Time to cook: 30-40 minutes
Servings: 12 slices

**Ingredients:**

- ½ cup butter, softened
- 2 eggs
- 1 tablespoon baking powder
- 1 cup buttermilk
- 1 cup stevia
- 2 cups all-purpose flour
- ½ teaspoon salt

**Directions:**

1. Get a 9-inch baking pan ready and preheat the oven to 350°F.
2. In a bowl, combine the dry ingredients.
3. In a different bowl, combine the stevia and butter. One by one, add the eggs, then thoroughly combine.
4. To make the mixture, add the flour and buttermilk in two separate batches and combine by gently folding.
5. Place the prepared dish in the oven and bake for 30 to 40 minutes, or until a toothpick inserted into the center comes out clean. Let it cool before serving.

**Nutritional Info:** Calories: 197; Fat: 8.8g; Carbs: 25.9g; Protein: 3.8g; Fiber: 0.6g

## White Chocolate Pudding

Time to prepare: 10 minutes
Time to cook: 5-8 minutes
Servings: 2-3

**Ingredients:**

- 2 tablespoon stevia
- A pinch of salt
- 1 large egg
- 2 tablespoon tapioca flour
- 1 cup non-dairy milk
- 3 oz unsweetened white chocolate chips

**Directions:**

1. In a pan, combine the dry ingredients. Whisk until smooth after adding the milk.
2. Stir the mixture frequently while cooking it over medium heat until it thickens and bubbles. Cook for two to three minutes at a low temperature. Get rid of the heat.
3. Add the egg mixture to the mixture and whisk. Allow it to simmer on low heat. You have two minutes to cook and stir. When melted, add the chocolate chip and stir.
4. Move to a bowl, thoroughly stir, and allow to cool for 15 minutes. Wrap in plastic wrap and serve warm or cold.

**Nutritional Info:** Calories: 387; Fat: 19.3g; Carbs: 41.5g; Protein: 8.3g; Fiber: 0.5g

## Peach N' Cherry Bake

Time to prepare: 10 minutes
Time to cook: 25-30 minutes
Servings: 4

**Ingredients:**

- 2 cups canned peaches, cut into small pieces
- 1 cup canned cherries, diced
- 2 tablespoon honey
- ½ cup all-purpose flour
- 2 tablespoon stevia
- 1 cup crushed cornflakes
- ¼ cup melted butter

**Directions:**

1. Set the oven's temperature to 350°F.
2. In a bowl, combine the butter, flour, sugar, and cornflakes to make a crumbly mixture. Spread the fruits on a baking sheet after mixing them with honey. Spread crumble evenly on top.

3. Bake for about 25 to 30 minutes, or until the topping becomes brown. Serve!

**Nutritional Info:** Calories: 295; Fat: 11.8g; Carbs: 45.7g; Protein: 2.6g; Fiber: 1.7g

## Banana And Apricot Ice Cream

Time to prepare: 10 minutes + freezing time
Time to cook: 0 minutes
Servings: 2

**Ingredients:**
- 1 cup ripe banana slices
- ½ cup canned apricot slices
- 1 cup non-dairy milk

**Directions:**
1. Use a blender to thoroughly combine all the ingredients.
2. To firm up more, serve right away or freeze in a silicon container, but not overnight.

**Nutritional Info:** Calories: 152; Fat: 1.7g; Carbs: 31g; Protein: 5.1g; Fiber: 1.9g

## Peach Mango Sorbet

Time to prepare: 10 minutes + freezing time
Time to cook: 0 minutes
Servings: 2

**Ingredients:**
- 1½ cups canned peaches
- 3-4 tablespoon stevia
- 1 cup canned mangoes/cherries

**Directions:**
1. Use a blender to thoroughly combine all the ingredients.
2. To firm up more, serve right away or freeze in a silicon container, but not overnight.

**Nutritional Info:** Calories: 81; Fat: 0.1g; Carbs: 21.3g; Protein: 0.6g; Fiber: 1g

## Peach Cherry Jam

Time to prepare: 10 minutes

Time to cook: 10 minutes
Servings: 1 cup

**Ingredients:**
- 2 cups peach, grated
- ½ cup of water
- 1 cup canned cherries
- 1 tablespoon honey

**Directions:**
1. In a pan of water, cook the peaches and cherries. until it turns into a thick liquid, simmer for 8 to 10 minutes.
2. Add the honey and whisk well. Let it cool, then put it in an airtight container and refrigerate it until you're ready to serve.

**Nutritional Info:** Calories: 53; Fat: 0g; Carbs: 10.4g; Protein: 0.4g; Fiber: 0.5g

## Frozen Strawberry-Peach Pops

Time to prepare: 10 minutes + freezing time
Time to cook: 10 minutes
Servings: 5

**Ingredients:**
- 1/2 cup stevia
- 6 oz canned strawberries
- 6 oz canned peaches
- 4 oz water
- 1 tablespoon lemon juice

**Directions:**
1. In a saucepan over medium heat, bring the water and stevia to a boil. Stirring frequently while the mixture simmers will cause the sugar to dissolve. Await cooling
2. Place all the ingredients in a blender and process until smooth. Strain the juice into a bowl using a fine-mesh strainer.
3. Fill your ice-pop molds with your juice, filling each one three-quarters of the way. Then, add your ice pop sticks and set the timer for at least five hours, or until the ice is solid. Serve!

**Nutritional Info:** Calories: 99; Fat: 0.1g; Carbs: 25g; Protein: 0.4g; Fiber: 1g

## Honey Lemonade Popsicles

Time to prepare: 10 minutes + freezing time
Time to cook: 0 minutes
Servings: 2

**Ingredients:**

- 1/2 cup honey
- 12 oz lemon juice
- 6 oz water

**Directions:**

1. In a saucepan over medium heat, combine the honey and water. Stirring occasionally, let the mixture simmer until the honey dissolves. Await cooling
2. Combine all of the ingredients in a spouted container. Fill each of the ice-pop molds with juice, about three-quarters full.
3. Include your ice pop sticks, and then place in the freezer for at least 5 hours, or until completely firm. Serve.

**Nutritional Info:** Calories: 292; Fat:0.4g; Carbs: 30.9g; Protein: 0.8g; Fiber: 0.6g

## Orange Strawberry Popsicles

Time to prepare: 10 minutes + freezing time
Time to cook: 0 minutes
Servings: 12 popsicles

**Ingredients:**

- 4 cups canned strawberry, hulled
- 2 cups orange juice
- 1 lime, juiced
- 1/4 cup honey

**Directions:**

1. Use your blender to thoroughly combine all the ingredients. The blended mixture should be strained through a fine-mesh strainer into a bowl.
2. Press the pulp to extract as much liquid as you can, then throw the pulp away. Fill each ice-pop mold with your juice, filling each one 3/4 full.
3. Include your ice pop sticks, and then place in the freezer for at least 5 hours, or until completely solid. Serve.

**Nutritional Info:** Calories: 57; Carbs: 14.3g; Fat: 0.2g; Protein: 0.6g; Fiber: 1.1g

## Melon Basil Moscow Mule Popsicles

Time to prepare: 10 minutes + freezing time
Time to cook: 0 minutes
Servings: 10 popsicles

**Ingredients:**

- 1 lb. cantaloupe, peeled, seeded, & chopped
- 7 mint leaves
- 4 oz water
- 4 oz limeade
- 16 oz ginger beer
- 2 oz simple syrup

**Directions:**

1. Use your blender to thoroughly combine all the ingredients. The blended mixture should be strained through a fine-mesh strainer into a bowl.
2. Press the pulp to extract as much liquid as you can, then throw the pulp away. Fill each ice-pop mold with your juice, filling each one 3/4 full.
3. Include your ice pop sticks, and then place in the freezer for at least 5 hours, or until completely solid. Serve.

**Nutritional Info:** Calories: 42; Fat: 0g; Carbs: 10.8g; Protein: 0.1g; Fiber: 0.2g

## Honeydew Mint Popsicles

Time to prepare: 10 minutes + freezing time
Time to cook: 0 minutes
Servings: 10 popsicles

**Ingredients:**

- ½ honeydew melon, peeled, seeded & cubed
- 1/3 cup granulated stevia
- 10 mint leaves
- 1 tablespoon lime juice

- 6 oz water

**Directions:**

1. Use your blender to thoroughly combine all the ingredients. The blended mixture should be strained through a fine-mesh strainer into a bowl.

2. Press the pulp to extract as much liquid as you can, then throw the pulp away. Fill each ice-pop mold with your juice, filling each one 3/4 full.

3. Include your ice pop sticks, and then place in the freezer for at least 5 hours, or until completely solid. Serve.

**Nutritional Info:** Calories: 35; Fat: 0g; Carbs: 9g; Protein: 0.1g; Fiber: 0.2g

## Basil Watermelon Popsicles

Time to prepare: 10 minutes + freezing time

Time to cook: 0 minutes

Servings: 12 popsicles

**Ingredients:**

- 1 lb. seedless watermelon, sliced
- 5 basil leaves
- 12 oz water
- 4 oz lime juice
- 1 oz honey

**Directions:**

1. Use your blender to thoroughly combine all the ingredients. The blended mixture should be strained through a fine-mesh strainer into a bowl.

2. Press the pulp to extract as much liquid as you can, then throw the pulp away. Fill each ice-pop mold with your juice, filling each one 3/4 full.

3. Include your ice pop sticks, and then place in the freezer for at least 5 hours, or until completely solid. Serve.

**Nutritional Info:** Calories: 16; Carbs: 4.4g; Fat: 0g; Protein: 0.2g; Fiber: 0.14g

## Orange Popsicles

Time to prepare: 10 minutes + freezing time

Time to cook: 0 minutes

Servings: 12 popsicles

**Ingredients:**

- 3 cups orange juice
- 1 lime, juiced

**Directions:**

1. Use your blender to thoroughly combine all the ingredients. The blended mixture should be strained through a fine-mesh strainer into a bowl.

2. Press the pulp to extract as much liquid as you can, then throw the pulp away. Fill each ice-pop mold with your juice, filling each one 3/4 full.

3. Include your ice pop sticks, and then place in the freezer for at least 5 hours, or until completely solid. Serve.

**Nutritional Info:** Calories: 29g; Fat: 0.1g; Carbs: 6.8g; Protein: 0.4g; Fiber: 0.1g

## Grapefruit Lemonade Popsicles

Time to prepare: 10 minutes + freezing time

Time to cook: 0 minutes

Servings: 12 popsicles

**Ingredients:**

- 1/4 cup honey
- 2 ½ cups grapefruit juice
- 12 oz lemon juice
- 6 oz water

**Directions:**

1. Use your blender to thoroughly combine all the ingredients. The blended mixture should be strained through a fine-mesh strainer into a bowl.

2. Press the pulp to extract as much liquid as you can, then throw the pulp away. Fill each ice-pop mold with your juice, filling each one 3/4 full.

3. Include your ice pop sticks, and then place in the freezer for at least 5 hours, or until completely solid. Serve.

**Nutritional Info:** Calories: 287; Fat: 2.5g; Carbs: 70g; Protein: 2.3g; Fiber: 1.5g

## Lemon Granita

Time to prepare: 5 minutes + freezing time

Time to cook: 5 minutes

Servings: 4

**Ingredients:**

- 3 lemons, juiced & zested
- 1/2 cup stevia
- 3 cups water

**Directions:**

1. Place the lemon zest and juice in a small saucepan. Over low heat, add the sugar and begin to boil. Within two minutes, simmer, then remove and add water.

2. Pour the mixture into an airtight container and strain through your fine sieve. Freeze for two hours.

3. Take it out, break up the ice with a fork, and then freeze it again for an additional hour.

**Nutritional Info:** Calories: 95; Fat: 0g; Carbs: 24g; Fiber: 0g; Protein: 0g

## Watermelon Ginger Juice

Time to prepare: 10 minutes
Time to cook: 0 minutes
Servings: 2
**Ingredients:**
- 4 cups seedless watermelon, cubed
- 1 teaspoon fresh ginger, peeled
- ½ tablespoon fresh lime juice

**Directions:**
1. Use a blender to thoroughly combine all the ingredients.
2. Strain the juice through your fine mesh strainer and pour it into your glasses. Serve right away.
**Nutritional Info:** Calories: 95; Fat: 0.5g; Carbs: 23.5g; Protein: 1.3g; Fiber: 1.9g

## Lemony Grapes Juice

Time to prepare: 10 minutes
Time to cook: 0 minutes
Servings: 3
**Ingredients:**
- 4 cups Seedless white grapes
- 2 tablespoon Fresh lemon juice

**Directions:**
1. Use a blender to thoroughly combine all the ingredients.
2. Strain the juice through your fine mesh strainer and pour it into your glasses. Serve right away.
**Nutritional Info:** Calories: 85; Fat: 0.5g; Carbs: 21.3g; Protein: 0.9g; Fiber: 1.1g

## Watermelon Plum Juice

Time to prepare: 10 minutes
Time to cook: 0 minutes
Servings: 2
**Ingredients:**
- 3 cups seedless watermelon, cut into chunks
- 4 plums, peeled, pitted & halved

- 6-8 ice cubes

**Directions:**
1. Use a blender to thoroughly combine all the ingredients.
2. Strain the juice through your fine mesh strainer and pour it into your glasses. Serve right away.
**Nutritional Info:** Calories: 129; Fat: 0.7g; Carbs: 33.1g; Protein: 2.3g; Fiber: 2.7g

## Watermelon Orange Juice

Time to prepare: 10 minutes
Time to cook: 0 minutes
Servings: 2
**Ingredients:**
- 1 cup fresh orange juice
- 4 cups seedless watermelon, chopped
- 5-6 fresh mint leaves
- 1-2 tablespoon honey

**Directions:**
1. Use a blender to thoroughly combine all the ingredients.
2. Strain the juice through your fine mesh strainer and pour it into your glasses. Serve right away.
**Nutritional Info:** Calories: 182; Fat: 0.7g; Carbs: 44.9g; Protein: 2.9g; Fiber: 1.9g

## Greens & Carrot Juice

Time to prepare: 10 minutes
Time to cook: 0 minutes
Servings: 2
**Ingredients:**
- 6 cups fresh spinach (if tolerated)
- 1 large carrot, peeled & chopped roughly
- 2 celery stalks
- 1 lemon
- 1 (1-inch) fresh ginger

**Directions:**

1. Use a blender to thoroughly combine all the ingredients.
2. Strain the juice through your fine mesh strainer and pour it into your glasses. Serve right away.
**Nutritional Info:** Calories: 36; Fat: 0.4g; Carbs: 7.1g Protein: 2.5g; Fiber: 2.7g

## Cucumber Grapefruit Juice

Time to prepare: 10 minutes
Time to cook: 0 minutes
Servings: 2
**Ingredients:**
- 4 seedless cucumbers, peeled & chopped
- 3 seedless grapefruits, peeled & sectioned
- 1 cup cold water

**Directions:**
1. Use a blender to thoroughly combine all the ingredients.
2. Strain the juice through your fine mesh strainer and pour it into your glasses. Serve right away.
**Nutritional Info:** Calories: 129; Fat: 0.7g; Carbs: 31.9g; Protein: 4.1g; Fiber: 3.1g

## Orange, Lemon & Lime Sports Drink

Time to prepare: 10 minutes
Time to cook: 0 minutes
Servings: 4
**Ingredients:**
- 4 ½ cups cold water
- 2 tablespoon fresh lime juice
- ¼ teaspoon salt
- 1/3 cup fresh orange juice
- 2 tablespoon fresh lemon juice
- 1 1/2 tablespoon honey

**Directions:**
1. Use a blender to thoroughly combine all the ingredients.
2. Strain the juice through your fine mesh strainer and pour it into your glasses. Serve right away.

**Nutritional Info:** Calories: 36; Fat: 0.1g; Carbs: 8.9g; Protein: 0.2g; Fiber: 0.1g

## Apple & Lime Sports Drink

Time to prepare: 10 minutes
Time to cook: 0 minutes
Servings: 4
**Ingredients:**
- 3 ½ cups spring water
- 1 teaspoon fresh lime juice
- 1/2 teaspoon sea salt
- 2 cups fresh apple juice
- 1 tablespoon honey

**Directions:**
1. In your pitcher, combine the water, lime juice, salt, apple juice, and honey.
2. Strain the juice through your fine mesh strainer and pour it into your large pitcher. Before serving, chill in the refrigerator.
**Nutritional Info:** Calories: 30; Fat: 0g; Carbs: 7.8g; Protein: 0.1g; Fiber: 0.1g

## Fresh Lemonade

Time to prepare: 10 minutes
Time to cook: 0 minutes
Servings: 4
**Ingredients:**
- 4 ½ cups Filtered water
- 3-4 drops of Stevia extract
- ¼ cup Fresh lemon juice

**Directions:**
1. In your pitcher, combine the stevia, water, and lemon juice.
2. Strain the juice through your fine mesh strainer and pour it into your large pitcher. Before serving, chill in the refrigerator.
**Nutritional Info:** Calories: 4; Fat: 0.1g; Carbs: 0.3g; Protein: 0.1g; Fiber: 0.1g

## Kiwi Juice

Time to prepare: 10 minutes

Time to cook: 0 minutes

Servings: 4

**Ingredients:**

- 4 medium kiwis, peeled & chopped
- 4 cups chilled filtered water

**Directions:**

1. Use a blender to thoroughly combine all the ingredients.

2. Strain the juice through your fine mesh strainer and pour it into your large pitcher. Before serving, chill in the refrigerator.

**Nutritional Info:** Calories: 93; Fat: 0.8g; Carbs: 22.3g; Protein: 1.7g; Fiber: 3g

## Nectarine Orange Juice

Time to prepare: 10 minutes

Time to cook: 0 minutes

Servings: 1

**Ingredients:**

- 2 nectarines, peeled, seeded
- 1 orange, juiced

**Directions:**

1. Use a blender to thoroughly combine all the ingredients.

2. Strain the juice through your fine mesh strainer and pour it into your large pitcher. Before serving, chill in the refrigerator.

**Nutritional Info:** Calories: 71; Fat: 0.4g; Carbs: 15.9g; Protein: 1.5g; Fiber: 0.5g

## Zucchini Cucumber Juice

Time to prepare: 10 minutes

Time to cook: 0 minutes

Servings: 1

**Ingredients:**

- 1 zucchini, peeled, seeded & sliced
- 2 cucumbers, peeled, seeded & sliced

**Directions:**

1. Use a blender to thoroughly combine all the ingredients.

2. Strain the juice through your fine mesh strainer and pour it into your glass. Serve!

**Nutritional Info:** Calories: 35; Fat: 0.4g; Carbs: 5.7g; Protein: 0.5g; Fiber: 0.8g

## Carrot Juice

Time to prepare: 10 minutes

Time to cook: 0 minutes

Servings: 1

**Ingredients:**

- 5-6 carrots, peeled & chopped
- ¼ cup coconut water

**Directions:**

1. Use a blender to thoroughly combine all the ingredients.

2. Strain the juice through your fine mesh strainer and pour it into your glass. Serve!

**Nutritional Info:** Calories: 50; Fat: 0.3g; Carbs: 11.5g; Protein: 1.2g; Fiber: 0.8g

## Peach Cherry Juice

Time to prepare: 10 minutes

Time to cook: 0 minutes

Servings: 2

**Ingredients:**

- ½ cup canned peach
- ½ cup canned cherry
- 1 cup water

**Directions:**

1. Use a blender to thoroughly combine all the ingredients.

2. Strain the juice through your fine mesh strainer and pour it into your glass. Serve!

**Nutritional Info:** Calories: 70; Fat: 0.1g; Carbs: 17.4g; Protein: 0.8g; Fiber: 1.5g

## Celery Juice

Time to prepare: 10 minutes

Time to cook: 0 minutes

Servings: 2

**Ingredients:**

- 8 celery stalks with leaves
- 2 tablespoon fresh ginger, peeled
- 1 lemon, peeled
- ½ cup filtered water
- Pinch of salt

**Directions:**
1. Use a blender to thoroughly combine all the ingredients.
2. Strain the juice through your fine mesh strainer and pour it into your glass. Serve!
**Nutritional Info:** Calories: 32; Fat: 0.5g; Carbs: 6.5g; Protein: 1g; Fiber: 2g

## Lychee Juice

Time to prepare: 10 minutes
Time to cook: 0 minutes
Servings: 2
**Ingredients:**
- 30 fresh lychees, peeled and pitted
- 1 cup of filtered water
- 2 tablespoon simple syrup

**Directions:**
1. Use a blender to thoroughly combine all the ingredients.
2. Strain the juice through your fine mesh strainer and pour it into your glass. Serve!
**Nutritional Info:** Calories: 159; Fat: 0.6g; Carbs: 40.6g; Protein: 1.2g; Fiber: 1.9g

## Peach Juice

Time to prepare: 10 minutes
Time to cook: 0 minutes
Servings: 2
**Ingredients:**
- 4 medium peaches, peeled, pitted & chopped
- 1 cup chilled water
- 1 tablespoon fresh lime juice

**Directions:**
1. Use a blender to thoroughly combine all the ingredients.
2. Strain the juice through your fine mesh strainer and pour it into your large pitcher. Before serving, chill in the refrigerator.
**Nutritional Info:** Calories: 119; Fat: 0.8g; Carbs: 28.1g; Protein: 2.8g; Fiber: 2.6g

## Plum Juice

Time to prepare: 10 minutes

Time to cook: 0 minutes
Servings: 2
**Ingredients:**
- 4 cups ripe plums, pitted and chopped
- 2 tablespoon maple syrup
- 1 cup of filtered water

**Directions:**
1. Use a blender to thoroughly combine all the ingredients.
2. Strain the juice through your fine mesh strainer and pour it into your large pitcher. Before serving, chill in the refrigerator.
**Nutritional Info:** Calories: 112; Fat: 0.4g; Carbs: 29.4g; Protein: 1g; Fiber: 1.8g

## Mango Juice

Time to prepare: 10 minutes
Time to cook: 0 minutes
Servings: 2
**Ingredients:**
- 4 cups mangoes, peeled, pitted & chopped
- 2 cups of filtered water

**Directions:**
1. Use a blender to thoroughly combine all the ingredients.
2. Strain the juice through your fine mesh strainer and pour it into your big pitcher. Before serving, chill in the refrigerator.
**Nutritional Info:** Calories: 99; Fat: 0.6g; Carbs: 24.7g; Protein: 1.4g; Fiber: 2.6g

## Carrot Orange Apple Tomato Juice

Time to prepare: 10 minutes
Time to cook: 0 minutes
Servings: 2
**Ingredients:**
- 1 medium yellow tomato, peeled, seeded & cut into wedges
- 1 orange, peeled, quartered
- 1 apple, peeled, cored, chopped
- 4 carrots, peeled, chopped
- 2 cups water

**Directions:**

1. Use a blender to thoroughly combine all the ingredients.

2. Strain the juice through your fine mesh strainer and pour it into your big pitcher. Before serving, chill in the refrigerator.

**Nutritional Info:** Calories: 111; Fat: 1g; Carbs: 24g; Protein: 2; Fiber: 1g

## Grapefruit Watermelon Juice

Time to prepare: 10 minutes
Time to cook: 0 minutes
Servings: 1

**Ingredients:**

- 1 grapefruit, peeled, seeded & sectioned
- 1 cup seedless watermelon, chunks

**Directions:**

1. Use a blender to thoroughly combine all the ingredients.

2. Strain the juice through your fine mesh strainer and pour it into your big pitcher. Before serving, chill in the refrigerator.

**Nutritional Info:** Calories: 108; Fat: 0.5g; Carbs: 27.3g; Protein: 2.6g; Fiber: 1.9g

## Carrot Lettuce Juice

Time to prepare: 10 minutes
Time to cook: 0 minutes
Servings: 1

**Ingredients:**

- 1 cup carrot, peeled & chopped
- 2 cups filtered water, + more if needed
- 1 cup lamb's lettuce

**Directions:**

1. Use a blender to thoroughly combine all the ingredients.

2. Strain the juice through your fine mesh strainer and pour it into your big pitcher. Before serving, chill in the refrigerator.

**Nutritional Info:** Calories: 107; Fat: 1g; Carbs: 21.4g; Protein: 3.3g; Fiber: 2.1g

## Apple Plum Juice

Time to prepare: 10 minutes
Time to cook: 0 minutes
Servings: 2

**Ingredients:**

- 1 apple, peeled, cored & sliced
- 2 cups coconut water
- 1 canned plum, peeled & deseeded

**Directions:**

1. Use a blender to thoroughly combine all the ingredients.

2. Strain the juice through your fine mesh strainer and pour it into your big pitcher. Before serving, chill in the refrigerator.

**Nutritional Info:** Calories: 112; Fat: 0.2g; Carbs: 28.3g; Protein: 0.9g; Fiber: 1.8g

## Cantaloupe Celery Juice

Time to prepare: 10 minutes
Time to cook: 0 minutes
Servings: 4

**Ingredients:**

- ½ of ripe cantaloupe, seeded & cut into chunks
- 4 celery stalks
- 1 large seedless cucumber, roughly chopped
- ½ of lemon, peeled

**Directions:**

1. Use a blender to thoroughly combine all the ingredients.

2. Strain the juice through your fine mesh strainer and pour it into your big pitcher. Before serving, chill in the refrigerator.

**Nutritional Info:** Calories: 42; Fat: 0.3g; Carbs: 10g; Protein: 1.6g; Fiber: 1.8g

## Celery & Carrot Juice

Time to prepare: 10 minutes
Time to cook: 0 minutes
Servings: 2

**Ingredients:**

- 4 celery stalks, roughly chopped
- 4 carrots, peeled & chopped roughly

- 1 tablespoon fresh lemon juice
- 1 cup of filtered water

**Directions:**

1. Use a blender to thoroughly combine all the ingredients.

2. Strain the juice through your fine mesh strainer and pour it into your big pitcher. Before serving, chill in the refrigerator.

**Nutritional Info:** Calories: 55; Fat: 0.1g; Carbs: 13g; Protein: 1.2g; Fiber: 3g

## Apple Cucumber Juice

Time to prepare: 10 minutes
Time to cook: 0 minutes
Servings: 2

**Ingredients:**

- 2 large seedless cucumbers, chopped
- 1 green apple, peeled, cored & chopped
- 1 cup water

**Directions:**

1. Use a blender to thoroughly combine all the ingredients.

2. Strain the juice through your fine mesh strainer and pour it into your big pitcher. Before serving, chill in the refrigerator.

**Nutritional Info:** Calories: 138; Fat: 1g; Carbs: 34.3g; Protein: 2.3g; Fiber: 2.2g

## Cucumber Celery Juice

Time to prepare: 10 minutes
Time to cook: 0 minutes
Servings: 2

**Ingredients:**

- 1 large seedless cucumber, roughly chopped
- 6 celery stalks, chopped
- 1 (1½-inch) piece of fresh ginger, peeled & roughly chopped
- 1 tablespoon fresh lemon juice
- ½ cup filtered water

**Directions:**

1. Use a blender to thoroughly combine all the ingredients.

2. Strain the juice through your fine mesh strainer and pour it into your big pitcher. Before serving, chill in the refrigerator.!

**Nutritional Info:** Calories: 46; Fat: 0.4g; Carbs: 9.2g; Protein: 41.6g; Fiber: 1.9g

## Simple Black Tea

Time to prepare: 10 minutes + steeping time
Time to cook: 5 minutes
Servings: 2

**Ingredients:**

- 2 cups of filtered water
- 1 teaspoon honey
- ½ teaspoon black tea leaves

**Directions:**

1. Put the water in a pan and bring it to a boil. Turn off the heat after adding the tea leaves.

2. Cover the pan right away and steep for 3 minutes. Once it has dissolved, add the honey and stir.

3. Pour the tea into glasses and serve right away.

**Nutritional Info:** Calories: 11; Fat: 0g; Carbs: 2.9g; Protein: 0g; Fiber: 0g

## Lemony Black Tea

Time to prepare: 10 minutes + steeping time
Time to cook: 0 minutes
Servings: 6

**Ingredients:**

- 1 tablespoon black tea leaves
- 1 cinnamon stick
- 1 lemon, sliced thinly
- 6 cups boiling water

**Directions:**

1. Fill a big teapot with the tea leaves, lemon slices, and cinnamon stick. Cover the teapot right away after adding boiling water to the contents.

2. Allow to steep for 5 minutes. Tea should be strained into glasses and served right away.

**Nutritional Info:** Calories: 1; Fat: 0g; Carbs: 0.2g; Protein: 0g; Fiber: 0g

## Chilled Green Tea

Time to prepare: 10 minutes + steeping time
Time to cook: 5 minutes
Servings: 6

**Ingredients:**
- 5 cups of filtered water
- ¼ cup fresh lemon juice
- ¼ cup honey
- 5 green tea bags
- ¼ cup fresh lime juice
- Ice cubes, as needed

**Directions:**
1. Fill your medium pan with 2 cups of water and bring it to a boil. After incorporating the tea bags, turn off the heat.
2. Cover the pan right away and steep for 3–4 minutes.
3. Gently press the tea bags on the pan with a large spoon to fully extract the tea. Take out the tea bags, then throw them away. Stir in the honey until it has dissolved.
4. In a large pitcher, blend the tea, lemon, and lime juices. Stir in the rest of the cold water after adding it. Tea should be poured into serving cups with ice cubes.

**Nutritional Info:** Calories: 46; Fat: 0.1g; Carbs: 12.2g; Protein: 0.1g; Fiber: 0.2g

## Warm Honey Green Tea

Time to prepare: 10 minutes + steeping time
Time to cook: 15 minutes
Servings: 4

**Ingredients:**
- 4 lemon's peel, cut into strips
- 4 lemon slices
- 4 orange's peel, cut into strips
- 4 cups of water
- 4 green tea bags
- 2 teaspoon honey

**Directions:**
1. Combine the strips and water in a pan. After bringing it to a boil, reduce the heat and simmer it for ten minutes. Remove the strips.
2. Include the tea bags and cover; allow the mixture to steep for 4-5 minutes. Remove the tea bags and mix in the honey. Serve with a lemon slice.

**Nutritional Info:** Calories 16; Fat 0.2g; Carbs 5g; Protein 0.2g; Fiber 0.6g

## Honey & Ginger Lemon Tea

Time to prepare: 5 minutes
Time to cook: 5 minutes
Servings: 1

**Ingredients:**
- 2 to 3 tablespoon lemon juice
- Hot water, as need
- Honey, to taste
- Fresh chopped ginger, to taste

**Directions:**
1. Put the water in a pan and bring it to a boil.
2. Fill your mug with the hot water and stir well before adding the remaining ingredients. Serve!

**Nutritional Info:** Calories 54; Fat 0.2g; Carbs 14g; Protein 0.2g; Fiber 0.2g

## Apple Cide Herbal Tea

Time to prepare: 10 minutes + steeping time
Time to cook: 0 minutes
Servings: 1

**Ingredients:**
- 2 tablespoon pure honey
- ¼ cup apple cider vinegar
- ¾ cup of herbal tea
- cayenne pepper, to taste
- hot water, as needed

**Directions:**

1. Pour the hot water and tea into your pitcher. Allow it to steep for four to five minutes.
2. After a thorough strain, add the remaining fixings. Stir well, then plate.
**Nutritional Info:** Calories 60; Fat 0.2g; Carbs 18.7g; Protein 0.1g; Fiber 1.2 g

## Peach Iced Tea

Time to prepare: 10 minutes + steeping time
Time to cook: 5 minutes
Servings: 2
**Ingredients:**
- 2 earl grey tea bag
- 4 cups of ice
- 2 cups of water

For the Peach Syrup:
- 2 tablespoon granulated stevia
- 1 ½ cups water
- 1 ½ cups diced peaches

**Directions:**
1. Steep the teas as directed on the package. The tea bags should be thrown away after 30 minutes in the refrigerator.
2. Place all the ingredients for the peach syrup in a blender and pulse to combine. For five minutes, simmer after adding it to a pan. Well, combine the tea after the straining and serve.
**Nutritional Info:** Calories 51; Fat 1g; Carbs 13g; Protein 1g; Fiber 1g

## Herbed Iced Tea

Time to prepare: 10 minutes + steeping time
Time to cook: 0 minutes
Servings: 8
**Ingredients:**
- 6 cups boiling water
- 2 cups fresh herbs
- 8 tea bags
- 4 cups of clear juice

**Directions:**

1. Follow the tea's package instructions for brewing. After 30 minutes in the refrigerator, throw away the tea bags.
2. In a blender, combine all the ingredients for the peach syrup by giving it a few pulses. It should then be simmered in a pan for five minutes. After straining, combine the tea and serve.
**Nutritional Info:** Calories 57; Fat 0.2g; Carbs 14g; Protein 0.1g; Fiber 1.2g

## Fruit-Infused Iced Green Tea

Time to prepare: 10 minutes + steeping time
Time to cook: 0 minutes
Servings: 8
**Ingredients:**
- 4 ½ cups boiling water
- 3 peaches, peeled, seeded & sliced thin
- 2 tablespoon honey
- 4 green tea bags
- 1 cup of blueberries (if tolerated)

**Directions:**
1. Follow the brewing directions on the tea's packaging. Discard the tea bags after 30 minutes in the fridge.
2. Pulse the ingredients for the peach syrup in a blender a few times to combine them. After that, it needs to simmer for five minutes in a pan. Combine the tea after filtering, then serve.
**Nutritional Info:** Calories 72; Fat 0.2g; Carbs 18.7g; Protein 0.1g; Fiber 1.2g

## Lemon Ginger Detox Tea

Time to prepare: 10 minutes + steeping time
Time to cook: 5 minutes
Servings: 2
**Ingredients:**
- ¼ teaspoon turmeric powder
- 2 cups water
- 1 (1 inch) of peeled ginger, sliced thinly

- ¼ teaspoon maple syrup
- 1 lemon, juiced
- Cayenne pepper, a pinch

**Directions:**

1. Place all the ingredients in a pan, stir well, and bring to a boil.

2. Turn off the heat and let the mixture steep for five minutes. and then serve.

**Nutritional Info:** Calories 12; Fat 0.2g; Carbs 2.8g; Protein 0.3g; Fiber 0.6g

## Melon Honey Green Tea

Time to prepare: 10 minutes
Time to cook: 0 minutes
Servings: 2

**Ingredients:**

- 1 bottle of unsweetened Honey Green Tea (not sweet)
- 6 chunks of honeydew melon, seeded & cut into small squares
- 15 fresh mint leaves

**Directions:**

1. Place all the ingredients in your bowl and mash with a spoon.

2. Combine well, filter, and serve.

**Nutritional Info:** Calories 72; Fat 0.2g; Carbs 1.1g; Protein 0.1g; Fiber 1.1g

## Iced Mint Green Tea

Time to prepare: 10 minutes + steeping time
Time to cook: 0 minutes
Servings: 3

**Ingredients:**

- Fresh mint leaves, as needed
- 3 green tea bags
- 1 lemon, thinly sliced
- 2 cups of boiling water

**Directions:**

1. Pour boiling water over the tea, remove the tea bags, and add the tea to a pot.

2. Add the lemon slices after allowing it to cool slightly. Allow your mint leaves to rest after you've added them. Serve.

**Nutritional Info:** Calories 0; Fat 0g; Carbs 0g; Protein 0g; Fiber 0g

## Apple Iced tea

Time to prepare: 10 minutes + steeping time
Time to cook: 0 minutes
Servings: 3

**Ingredients:**

- 4 cups of boiling water
- 1 lemon, thinly sliced
- 2 cinnamon sticks
- 4 cups of clear apple juice
- 2 English breakfast tea bags
- 1 red apple, peeled, cored & thinly sliced
- Honey, to taste

**Directions:**

1. Add the tea to a saucepan, then pour boiling water over it after removing the tea bags.

2. After letting it somewhat cool, add the lemon slices. After adding the mint leaves, give them time to rest. Serve.

**Nutritional Info:** Calories 72; Fat 0.2g; Carbs 18.7g; Protein 0.1g; Fiber 1.2g

## The All-Fix Tea

Time to prepare: 10 minutes + steeping time
Time to cook: 0 minutes
Servings: 1

**Ingredients:**

- 1 tablespoon honey
- 1" of sliced fresh ginger
- 1 small stick of cinnamon
- 1 sliced clove of garlic (if tolerated)
- Juice of 1/2 lemon

**Directions:**

1. After removing the tea bags, add the tea to a saucepan and then pour boiling water over it.

2. Add the lemon slices after allowing it to slightly cool. Give the mint leaves some

time to rest after you've added them. Serve.

**Nutritional Info:** Calories 65; Fat 0.2g; Carbs 11g; Protein 0.1g; Fiber 1g

## Immune Booster Herbal Tea

Time to prepare: 10 minutes + steeping time
Time to cook: 0 minutes
Servings: 1

**Ingredients:**
- 1 tablespoon dried elderberries
- 1 tablespoon dried echinacea flowers & leaves
- 1 tablespoon dried ginger root
- 1 tablespoon dried rose hips
- 1 tablespoon dried astragalus
- 1 cup boiling water
- Honey, as needed

**Directions:**
1. Combine all the ingredients in an airtight container. Mix well, then store in a dry, cool environment.
2. Pour 1 tablespoon of the mixture into a mug, top it off with boiling water, and let it steep for at least 30 minutes.
3. After a thorough straining, taste-test and add honey as desired. Serve.

**Nutritional Info:** Calories 65; Fat 0.2g; Carbs 11g; Protein 0.2g; Fiber 1.1g

## NyQuell Herbal Tea

Time to prepare: 10 minutes + steeping time
Time to cook: 0 minutes
Servings: 1-2

**Ingredients:**
- 1 tablespoon dried valerian root
- 1 tablespoon dried peppermint leaf
- 1 tablespoon dried chamomile flower
- 1 tablespoon dried licorice root
- 1-2 cups boiling water
- Honey, as needed

**Directions:**

1. Combine all the ingredients in an airtight container. Mix well, then store in a dry, cool environment.
2. To prepare one cup of tea, place one tablespoon of the mixture in a mug, top with boiling water, and steep for 30 minutes or longer. Add honey to your taste after a thorough straining. Serve.

**Nutritional Info:** Calories 67; Fat 0.3g; Carbs 11g; Protein 0.1g; Fiber 1.1g

## Mint & Ginger Iced Green Tea

Time to prepare: 10 minutes + steeping time
Time to cook: 5 minutes
Servings: 4

**Ingredients:**
- ¼ cup peeled ginger, sliced
- 1/3 cup honey
- 3-6 green tea bags
- 1 lemon, divided
- 6 cups water
- 1/2 cup of mint leaves

**Directions:**
1. Put water and ginger in your pot. Add the mint and tea bags after allowing it to boil.
2. After 15 minutes of steeping, strain well and stir in the honey. Offer cold.

**Nutritional Info:** Calories 75; Fat 0.2g; Carbs 18.7g; Protein 0.1g; Fiber 1.2g

## Strawberry-Basil Iced Tea

Time to prepare: 10 minutes + steeping time
Time to cook: 5 minutes
Servings: 8

**Ingredients:**
- 1 lb. strawberries, trimmed & cut into fours
- 1 cup of fresh basil
- 4 cups of water or more
- 8 black-tea bags
- 3/4 cup stevia

- Ice, for serving

**Directions:**

1. Add water to a pan and bring it to a boil. After adding tea bags, let it steep for five minutes.

2. Combine the stevia and water in another saucepan. Cook while stirring constantly over low heat until the sugar melts.

3. Add the basil after turning the heat off. Give it ten minutes to relax. Combine thoroughly with the strawberries after adding them. Give it 25 minutes to relax.

4. Combine the strawberries and tea, then refrigerate for a few hours to let the flavors blend. After straining, serve cold.

**Nutritional Info:** Calories 79; Fat 0.2g; Carbs 19g; Protein 0.1g; Fiber 1g

### Hibiscus-Mint Iced Tea

Time to prepare: 10 minutes + steeping time

Time to cook: 0 minutes

Servings: 8

**Ingredients:**

- 4 cups boiling water
- 4 hibiscus tea bags
- 2 cups cold water
- 1/2 cup of fresh mint leaves
- 2 cups apple juice

**Directions:**

1. Fill a pot with boiling water, tea bags, and mint leaves. Allow it to steep for ten minutes.

2. Remove the tea and mint bags. Apple juice and cold water should be added. Mix thoroughly, then plate.

**Nutritional Info:** Calories 81; Fat 0.2g; Carbs 12g; Protein 1g; Fiber 1.3g

### Peppermint Tea

Time to prepare: 10 minutes + steeping time

Time to cook: 5 minutes

Servings: 2

**Ingredients:**

- 2-3 cups of water
- 1 tablespoon fresh peppermint leaves, crushed
- 3-4 herbal tea bags
- 1 tablespoon oregano leaves, crushed

**Directions:**

1. In a saucepan, bring the water to a boil before adding the oregano, tea bags, and peppermint leaves.

2. Cover and steep for five to ten minutes. Serve the tea warm after straining.

**Nutritional Info:** Calories: 5; Fat: 0.3g; Carbs: 0.5g; Protein: 0.3g; Fiber: 0.2g

### Sage Rosemary Tea

Time to prepare: 10 minutes + steeping time

Time to cook: 5 minutes

Servings: 2

**Ingredients:**

- 2-3 cups of water
- 2 tablespoon fresh sage leaves, crushed
- 1 tablespoon fresh rosemary leaves, crushed

**Directions:**

1. Fill a pot with water, then bring it to a boil. For 10 minutes, remove, cover, and steep.

2. Strain the tea, then warmly serve.

**Nutritional Info:** Calories: 2; Fat: 0.3g; Carbs: 1.4g; Protein: 0.3g; Fiber: 0.4g

### Sweet Melon Zucchini Smoothie

Time to prepare: 10 minutes

Time to cook: 0 minutes

Servings: 1

**Ingredients:**

- 1 cup sweet melon, seeded & sliced
- 1 cup of filtered water
- 1 zucchini, peeled, seeded & sliced
- A dash of honey to taste

**Directions:**

1. Use a blender to thoroughly combine all the ingredients.
2. Dish out and savor!

**Nutritional Info:** Calories: 62; Fat: 0.4g; Carbs: 14.8g; Protein: 1.8g; Fiber: 1.7g

## Mint Grape Smoothie

Time to prepare: 10 minutes
Time to cook: 0 minutes
Servings: 1
**Ingredients:**
- 1 cup seedless grapes
- 4-5 fresh mint leaves
- 1 cup coconut/plain water

**Directions:**
1. Use a blender to thoroughly combine all the ingredients.
2. Dish out and savor!

**Nutritional Info:** Calories: 104; Fat: 0.3g; Carbs: 27g; Protein: 1.1g; Fiber: 1.4g

## Avocado Passion Smoothie

Time to prepare: 10 minutes
Time to cook: 0 minutes
Servings: 2
**Ingredients:**
- 1 teaspoon apple butter
- ¼ cup scooped avocado (if tolerated)
- 1 cup coconut/regular water
- 1 cup passionfruit, deseeded
- 1 teaspoon whey/soy protein powder
- A few canned cherries
- Ice cubes, as needed

**Directions:**
1. Use a blender to thoroughly combine all the ingredients.
2. Dish out and savor!

**Nutritional Info:** Calories: 112; Fat: 3g; Carbs: 20.4g; Protein: 1.3g; Fiber: 1.4g

## Papaya Carrot Smoothie

Time to prepare: 10 minutes
Time to cook: 0 minutes
Servings: 1
**Ingredients:**
- 1 cup papaya, pitted
- ½ -¾ cup low-fat milk
- ½ cup canned carrot, peeled

**Directions:**
1. Use a blender to thoroughly combine all the ingredients.
2. Dish out and savor!

**Nutritional Info:** Calories: 186; Fat: 2.3g; Carbs: 34.2g; Protein: 6.8g; Fiber: 2.3g

## Papaya-Mango Smoothie

Time to prepare: 5 minutes
Time to cook: 0 minutes
Servings: 2
**Ingredients:**
- 1 cup mango, diced
- 1 cup papaya chunks
- 1 cup almond milk
- 1 tablespoon honey or maple syrup

**Directions:**
1. Use a blender to thoroughly combine all the ingredients.
2. Dish out and savor!

**Nutritional Info:** Calories: 554; Fat: 32g; Carbs: 14g; Protein: 50g; Fiber: 2g

## Cantaloupe Smoothie

Time to prepare: 5 minutes
Time to cook: 0 minutes
Servings: 2
**Ingredients:**
- 1 cup cantaloupe, diced
- ½ cup lactose-free yogurt
- ½ cup orange juice
- 1 tablespoon honey or maple syrup
- 2 ice cubes

**Directions:**
1. Use a blender to thoroughly combine all the ingredients.
2. Dish out and savor!

**Nutritional Info:** Calories: 179; Fat: 13g; Carbs: 6g; Protein: 10g; Fiber: 1g

## Cantaloupe-Mix Smoothie

Time to prepare: 5 minutes
Time to cook: 0 minutes
Servings: 2
**Ingredients:**

- 1 cup cantaloupe, diced
- ½ cup mango, diced
- ½ cup almond milk
- ½ cup orange juice
- 2 tablespoon lemon juice
- 1 tablespoon honey or maple syrup
- 2 ice cubes

**Directions:**
1. Use a blender to thoroughly combine all the ingredients.
2. Dish out and savor!
**Nutritional Info:** Calories: 329; Fat: 17g; Carbs: 9g; Protein: 37g; Fiber: 2.9g

## Applesauce-Avocado Smoothie

Time to prepare: 5 minutes
Time to cook: 0 minutes
Servings: 1
**Ingredients:**

- 1 cup unsweetened almond milk
- ½ avocado, pitted & sliced
- ½ cup applesauce
- ¼ teaspoon ground cinnamon
- ½ cup ice
- ½ teaspoon stevia or 1 tablespoon honey for sweetness (optional)

**Directions:**
1. Use a blender to thoroughly combine all the ingredients.
2. Dish out and savor!
**Nutritional Info:** Calories: 270; Fat: 11g, Carbs: 4g; Protein: 39g; Fiber: 1g

## Orange Banana Smoothie

Time to prepare: 5 minutes
Time to cook: 2 minutes

Servings: 2
**Ingredients:**

- 1 large banana, sliced
- ¾ cup orange juice
- ¼ cup almond milk
- ¼ teaspoon maple syrup

**Directions:**
1. Use a blender to thoroughly combine all the ingredients.
2. Dish out and savor!
**Nutritional Info:** Calories: 120; Fat: 2g; Carbs: 30g; Protein: 2g; Fiber: 2g

## Ginger Turmeric Smoothie

Time to prepare: 5 minutes
Time to cook: 0 minutes
Servings: 2
**Ingredients:**

- 1 banana
- 1 tablespoon cashew nut butter
- 1 tablespoon ground turmeric
- 2 thumb-size pieces of ginger, chopped finely & peeled
- 1 cup almond milk

**Directions:**
1. Use a blender to thoroughly combine all the ingredients.
2. Dish out and savor!
**Nutritional Info:** Calories: 72; Fat: 0g; Carbs: 0g, Protein: 5g; Fiber: 2.5g

## Pineapple Green Smoothie

Time to prepare: 5 minutes
Time to cook: 0 minutes
Servings: 2
**Ingredients:**

- 1 cup non-dairy milk
- 1 frozen banana, sliced
- 1 cup baby spinach (if tolerated)
- 1 cup pineapple chunks (fresh or frozen)

**Directions:**
1. Use a blender to thoroughly combine all the ingredients.

2. Dish out and savor!
**Nutritional Info:** Calories: 131; Fat: 2g; Carbs: 28g; Protein: 1g; Fiber: 1.7g

## Vanilla Shake

Time to prepare: 5 minutes
Time to cook: 0 minutes
Servings: 1
**Ingredients:**
- ¼ cup non-dairy yogurt
- ¼ cup vanilla ice cream
- ¼ prepared Jell-O

**Directions:**
1. Use a blender to thoroughly combine all the ingredients.
2. Dish out and savor!

**Nutritional Info:** Calories: 144; Fat: 12g; Carbs: 21g; Protein: 5g; Fiber: 0g

## Lemon-Apple-Honey Smoothie

Time to prepare: 10 minutes
Time to cook: 0 minutes
Servings: 4
**Ingredients:**
- ¼ cup lemon juice
- ½ cup apple juice
- 1 apple, peeled & cored
- 1 banana, sliced
- 2 to 3 teaspoon honey
- 1 cup vanilla yogurt, frozen

**Directions:**
1. Use a blender to thoroughly combine all the ingredients.
2. Dish out and savor!
**Nutritional Info:** Calories: 170; Fat: 7g; Carbs: 38g; Protein: 2g; Fiber: 1.3g

## Pina Colada Smoothie

Time to prepare: 5 minutes
Time to cook: 0 minutes
Servings: 2
**Ingredients:**
- 1 cup pineapple, canned

- 1 teaspoon Stevia or another sweetener
- 1 cup tofu, firm
- ½ cup of pineapple juice, unsweetened

**Directions:**
1. Use a blender to thoroughly combine all the ingredients.
2. Dish out and savor!
**Nutritional Info:** Calories: 189; Fat: 5g; Carbs: 32g; Protein: 13.4g; Fiber: 1.8g

## Peach Rice Smoothie

Time to prepare: 10 minutes
Time to cook: 0 minutes
Servings: 2
**Ingredients:**
- 2 peaches, peeled
- 4 tablespoon rice flakes
- 2 cups almond milk
- 1 teaspoon ginger, peeled & freshly minced
- 1 teaspoon cinnamon

**Directions:**
1. Use a blender to thoroughly combine all the ingredients.
2. Dish out and savor!
**Nutritional Info:** Calories: 212; Fat: 5.8g; Carbs: 35g; Protein: 11.6g; Fiber: 2.2g

## Banana Cherry Smoothie

Time to prepare: 10 minutes
Time to cook: 0 minutes
Servings: 2
**Ingredients:**
- 1 large banana cubed
- 2 cup milk
- ½ cup canned cherries

**Directions:**
1. Use a blender to thoroughly combine all the ingredients.
2. Dish out and savor!

**Nutritional Info:** Calories: 185; Fat: 2.7g; Carbs: 33g; Protein: 9.4g; Fiber: 2.2g

## Apple Butter Melon Smoothie

Time to prepare: 10 minutes
Time to cook: 0 minutes
Servings: 2
**Ingredients:**
- 1 cup cantaloupe or other melon, cubed
- 1 tablespoon apple butter
- 2 tablespoon canned cherries
- 1 cup almond milk

**Directions:**
1. Use a blender to thoroughly combine all the ingredients.
2. Dish out and savor!

**Nutritional Info:** Calories: 203; Fat: 12.5g; Carbs: 36.6g; Protein: 10g; Fiber: 1.1g

## Carrot Plum Zucchini Smoothie

Time to prepare: 10 minutes
Time to cook: 0 minutes
Servings: 2
**Ingredients:**
- 1 cup canned chopped carrots, peeled
- 1 tablespoon honey
- 1 canned plum or another low-fiber fruit
- 1 medium zucchini, peeled
- 1 to 1½ cup almond milk

**Directions:**
1. Use a blender to thoroughly combine all the ingredients.
2. Dish out and savor!

**Nutritional Info:** Calories: 140; Fat: 2.3g; Carbs: 26.8g; Protein: 5g; Fiber: 2.1g.

## CONCLUSION

Now, particularly if you have ulcerative colitis, figuring out which foods would best nourish your body is not difficult. In order to improve your gut health and alleviate some of the symptoms of the condition, such as diarrhea and constipation, we have provided you with recipes that are low in fiber and residue. This cookbook contains simple dishes that require little cleaning and preparation. The recipes may also be followed by those on a limited diet, allowing you to continue eating the things you adore while still feeling filled and healthy. This cookbook's recipes provide a guide on how to approach your food in a manner that relieves your symptoms and promotes your health.

You may need to avoid certain foods or take additional care to make sure you are getting adequate nutrients in order to reduce your symptoms. You may even need to change your diet in certain circumstances to cut out particular foods or food categories. If so, you may adjust your diet using the recipes in this cookbook so that you can still enjoy your favorite foods without having to fully give them up.

You'll experience a sense of nourishment and restoration as a result, which will make it easier for you to control your symptoms. You will be better able to make choices that promote your health after you comprehend how food impacts your body.

# -THE END-

Made in United States
Troutdale, OR
06/06/2023

10465780R00081